CATCHING
HOMELESSNESS

JOSEPHINE ENSIGN

CATCHING HOMELESSNESS

A Nurse's Story of Falling Through the Safety Net

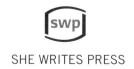

SHE WRITES PRESS

Published 2016
Printed in the United States of America
Print ISBN: 978-1-63152-117-1
E-ISBN: 978-1-63152-118-8
Library of Congress Control Number: 2016937782

For information, address:
She Writes Press
1563 Solano Ave #546
Berkeley, CA 94707

Cover design © Rebecca Lown
Interior design © Tabitha Lahr

She Writes Press is a division of SparkPoint Studio, LLC.

Portions of the book have appeared in print in different forms:

"First Families" was published as "Gone South" in *Silk Road*, Vol 6.1, Spring 2011.

"Homeless Ghosts" was published in University of Iowa's *The Examined Life Journal*, Issue 2.1, Fall 2012.

"Next of Kin" was published in the anthology *I Wasn't Strong Like This When I Started Out: True Stories of Becoming a Nurse*, edited by Lee Gutkind, In Fact Books, 2013.

Parts of "Catching Homelessness" were published as "No Place Like Home(less)" in *Pulse: Voices from the Heart of Medicine* magazine, May 30, 2014.

"Greyhound Therapy" was published in *Front Porch Journal*, Issue 32, Spring 2016.

In memory of my mother,
Ruth Singley Ensign (1923–2008)

Most of us live homeless, in the neighborhood of our true selves.
—Rachel Naomi Remen

CONTENTS

Author's Note

A FEW YEARS AGO, while working with Public Health–
Seattle & King County on a medical respite project for
homeless youth, my own homeless shadow resurfaced. I
was in downtown Seattle at the YWCA women's shelter,
waiting inside the front lobby for the rest of our group to
arrive. We were scheduled to have a tour of the facility to
see how they ran their medical respite program. I'd taken
the city bus and had purposefully dressed down in jeans, a
sweater, and a raincoat. It was late afternoon, raining outside, and I saw soliciting, pimping, prostituting, and drug
dealing happening on the sidewalk in front of the shelter.
The members of my medical respite group were buzzed in
the front door. At the same time, a homeless woman resi-
dent walked up to me and asked, "Did you stay at a hotel
last night on Aurora instead of here again?" Aurora Avenue is one of Seattle's main prostitution areas.

I looked up at her in alarm. "I'm sorry. You must have me mixed up with someone else. I'm not staying here, I'm just visiting."

The people in my group overheard this interchange. Later, they teased me about it, saying how preposterous it was. I was a university professor, for God's sake! There was no way I could be homeless, much less a homeless prostitute. But I couldn't shake the feeling that my cover had been blown, that I'd been found out, that my homeless shadow was showing. You were homeless—why? What was wrong with you? Those are the questions people ask me—or want to ask me—whenever they discover I was homeless. Coming out of the closet about my own homelessness was never an option for me. It could derail my career, hurt my family, and marginalize me even more. It was largely why I had moved across the country to Seattle, to escape the memories of having been homeless in my hometown of Richmond, Virginia. But standing there in the YWCA shelter, I recognized the irony—and the hypocrisy—embedded in my reaction to the woman's question. Here I was an outspoken advocate for people who were homeless, while secretly judging them, and by extension, judging myself.

Homelessness is exhausting and soul sucking. Homelessness has marked me. Like the star-shaped surgery scars on my belly, the body harbors secrets. Homelessness is a type of deep illness, a term coined by sociologist Arthur Frank for an illness that leaves you feeling dislocated, an illness that casts a shadow over your life. That shadow never completely goes away. At some point it was time to acknowledge my homeless shadow, time to remember.

This book is the result of my acknowledging and remembering. It is the story of my experiences with homelessness, both as a nurse practitioner working with homeless people, and as a homeless person. The stories in *Catching Homelessness* are about events that have happened to me through my work with homeless people. The stories are all factual in that they actually happened. My perception of them at the time of the events and my memories of them inform the stories. Many of my interactions with people in these stories were within an ongoing professional relationship. Since I recount stories of specific patients I worked with, out of ethical and legal obligations I have altered some biographical details and changed names in order to protect their identities. I have not changed the names of coworkers and friends, except where indicated.

I have kept detailed journals, both personal and work-related, throughout my life. These were invaluable resources for writing this book. Because I have a background and training in anthropology, my work-related journals were written as expanded field notes. In my journals I recorded patient stories, direct quotes, profiles, and personality quirks of coworkers, as well as my reflections on my actions and on events with which I was involved. I kept copies of my detailed monthly and year-end clinic statistics, narrative reports, and letters that I submitted to the CrossOver Clinic board of directors, for whom I worked; these became sources of information for sections of this book. I also drew upon archived newspaper articles, mainly from *The Richmond Times-Dispatch*, the leading newspaper in Richmond at the time, and currently the city's only major newspaper. For some chapters, I relied on interviews with people working with homeless people in Richmond, site visits, and reports (past and present) on homelessness in Richmond and in Virginia, as well as nationally. In the appendices I include a list of the main references I consulted while writing this book.

I use terms for race or ethnicity based on the commonly

accepted terms during the time period for which I am writing, or the terms preferred by the people I am writing about. Hence, I use "black" or "African-American," "Native American" or "American Indian" depending on the context. Other terms, such as "mentally retarded" or "developmentally disabled," I use based on accepted terminology within the US medical and legal realms of a particular time period.

Stories analyze us if we pay attention to what attracts or repels us while reading or hearing the stories, and if we reflect on why that is so. Stories we understand are stories we easily forget. Perhaps that is why the stories I recount in this book are the ones that most vividly survived for me. I don't completely understand them. Even after writing them—an act that brings some coherence—they keep their secrets.

Catching Homelessness is about what people who have experienced homelessness can teach us about our society and ourselves. My aim is to provide a framework for the empathy necessary to create positive change for people pushed to the margins. By illuminating the margins, we can see more of the truth about our society's core, and about ourselves.

CHAPTER ONE:

Next of Kin

IT WAS A COLD APRIL day in 1989 in my hometown of Richmond, Virginia. I was at my first funeral. Standing graveside, I wondered why I had never been to a funeral before. I was about to turn twenty-nine years old; surely most people my age had been to a funeral.

The rain beat down hard and fast around me, sending echoes under the canvas tarp and out across the fields of tombstones. The words of the black Baptist preacher faltered, out of synch with the rhythm of the rain. He sucked in a lungful of biting air and led us in the Lord's Prayer. When he got to, "And forgive us our debts . . . ," he straightened his spine and arched his head back, with his eyes tightly closed and hands uplifted. A gray casket lay at his feet. Several flowered wreaths were strewn across the top, and some were standing in front on spindly wire legs. A thin black woman sat in a metal, folding chair near the casket. She wore a large-brimmed black hat. A row of large black women stood like sentinels behind her.

Huddled in clusters under the tarp stood fifteen or so black people, mostly women, a few uncomfortable-looking men, and one small boy dressed in a fedora and oversized raincoat, the sleeves hanging limply to his knees. He kept fidgeting, pushing the hat back off his face, and twisting around to stare at me with large dark eyes heavily fringed with long lashes. I stood under the outer edge of the canvas tarp, one of two white faces in the crowd, the only person with blue eyes, and the only person not wearing black. Instead, I was wearing a tan trench coat, belted tightly over my bright-blue knit dress. I hadn't realized that people still wore black to funerals. I was worried I was offending the family. The other white face was of the older social worker standing beside me. She had arranged the funeral.

While half-listening to the preacher, I tried to figure out who the seated woman was. Besides the casket, the woman was the center of this gathering; the preacher was more of a prop, like the flower wreaths. The social worker saw me gazing at the seated woman, leaned toward me, and whispered, "That's Lee's mother. He hadn't seen her in fifteen years. She got here too late."

I nodded and hugged my arms tighter, closing my coat. The wind had picked up and was blowing cold rain under the tarp. A flowered wreath toppled over in a gust, but no one picked it up.

Lee was thirty-eight years old and homeless; he'd been a patient of mine for the past three years. He had died of AIDS the week before and now his body was in the casket, ready to be buried.

I worked as a nurse practitioner at the CrossOver Clinic, part of a multiservice center for homeless people called the

Richmond Street Center. Located in downtown Richmond, the Street Center housed a shelter, soup kitchen, laundry and shower services, and the offices of many social workers, including the one who had arranged Lee's funeral. I gazed out over the soft contours of the wet, gray graveyard. I felt like an intruder in a private and complicated grief for a part of a man I hadn't known.

There were ten or so parked cars lined up on the road nearby, and a large orange tractor revving its engines to the left of us a few yards away. It dangled a concrete casket encasement in front, waiting impatiently to finish its business of burying Lee. I wondered if they were more respectful at private cemeteries. Lee was being buried in the Potter's Field section of the city-run Oakwood Cemetery, next to the all-black Evergreen Cemetery, overgrown with ivy, where human bones tumbled out of disintegrating mausoleums. At least this cemetery was well-maintained, probably because over seventeen thousand Confederate soldiers were buried here. Oakwood was the Civil War burial site for soldiers who died at the nearby Chimborazo Hospital of the Confederate Army. One of the remaining stone buildings of the hospital was now a museum on a high bluff overlooking the James River, just south of where we stood. The Confederate soldiers' graves were located near the entrance of the cemetery, with short white uniform gravestones marching over the hill, some marked with small Confederate flags. It struck me for the first time—as more than an abstract idea—that even in death, people are divided.

As a nurse, I had seen death many times, had washed newly dead people in the hospital, done their paperwork, and zipped them into body bags. This was different. I was seeing where the body went after the body bag, after the morgue, after the funeral home. And I was seeing Lee's family for the first time. He had never mentioned them, never asked for them in his final days. He died alone. They were black, I was white, and we were in the capital of the Confederacy, where it's not easy to be color-blind.

As the preacher wrapped up Lee's graveside service with the last "Amen!" the social worker whispered to me, "I've got to go pay the preacher. Thanks for coming, Jo. Lee was a great guy." I nodded as she walked away.

Lee's mother leaned forward and placed a hand on Lee's casket. Her shoulders convulsed with sobs.

I hesitated, wondering if I should stay and introduce myself to Lee's family, tell them how sorry I was that he died. But Lee's mother was still crying and I was cold and wet, so I walked back to my car. I drove slowly through the winding, pot-holed cemetery road, over the one-lane bridge crossing the ravine, and out past the graves of the Confederate soldiers. As I drove home, I thought back over my years of working with Lee.

I had first met Lee on a snowy December morning three years before. He walked into the Street Center Clinic, coughing, and grinning widely at me between coughs as he unwrapped a large scarf from around his face. His cough was a deep rattle, surprisingly loud coming from such a small-framed man. Lee had a boyish round face, burnished dark skin, and large brown eyes framed by lush curled lashes. He was wearing an old green Army coat with a matted fake fur fringed hood and an orange watch cap pulled down tightly over his closely cropped hair.

"Morning, nurse. They sent me over here from the job site 'cause they're tired of hearing me cough. You got anything for it?" He pulled the hat off his head, kneading his hair back into place with his knuckles.

"Sure, come on in and have a seat. Let me check you

out first. Take a listen to your lungs and see what I can do." I gestured to the black padded metal chair sitting against one wall inside my office.

I had been at the Street Center Clinic eight months, working out of an eight-by-ten-foot one-room clinic in a corner of the third and topmost floor of the flat-roofed red-brick building. The Street Center was thick-walled, dank, and cavernous. It was located in the armpit of town, on the border between Monroe Ward, Gamble's Hill, and Oregon Hill near the James River, upriver from Church Hill and the Oakwood Cemetery. Built on land that had been the old city dump, the Street Center building had been a gas meter repair shop for the city, as well as a storage unit for abandoned bicycles. The city donated the building as a way to appease the downtown merchants who wanted to get the street people, the visible homeless, away from their struggling businesses. Empty lots surrounded the Street Center on three sides. Kudzu vines draped over trees and telephone poles, forming a convenient curtain to block the public's view of the ugly, forbidding-looking building.

The Street Center was located at the corner of Belvidere and Canal Streets, with the main entrance on Canal Street. The building was flush with the cracked sidewalk. Across Canal Street from the Street Center was the recessed and fenced-off Downtown Expressway, with its roar of speeding cars. Belvidere Street, a busy four-lane highway that ran north to south, was part of US Route 301 extending down to Sarasota, Florida, and up to Delaware. Across Belvidere from the Street Center was a 7-Eleven that sold cigarettes, cheap beer, and flavored wine like Boone's Farm, Thunderbird, and Wild Irish Rose, all popular with the Street Center clientele. South of the Street Center were the hulking brick buildings and serpentine razor wire of the Virginia Penitentiary. Just to the west was Hollywood Cemetery, where a relative of mine, Jefferson Davis, and eighteen thousand Confederate soldiers lay buried. In the block north of our building was a Hostess Twinkie factory. The sweet buttery smell of the factory mingled with the acrid smells of the Street Center: damp oil-stained concrete, souring unwashed bodies, old urine, and stale cigarette smoke.

I worked alone in the clinic and was the only health care provider at the Street Center during the week. Volunteer physicians came on Saturdays to see the more medically complex patients. My clinic office in the Street Center had a built-in white Formica countertop along one wall, with a small sink in the corner, all held up by small file cabinets. A large mustard-yellow metal desk took up most of the floor space. It was covered by large hardbound medical reference books, and had a locked drawer where I stored medications such as antibiotics, fungal skin creams, and cough medicine. I had no exam table when I first started out, so patients sat on the padded metal chair beside the door. The clinic had West-facing windows, which were loose single panes in old rusting metal frames. The windowpanes rattled in the wind, which was blowing wildly on the December day I first met Lee. The building's heating system barely worked, so I was wearing my orange down coat over my white lab coat. Both coats were open over my expanding belly. I was four months pregnant with my first child. The room's whitewashed walls blazed even whiter under the bank of fluorescent ceiling lights, lights which supposedly killed tuberculosis germs. That's what I'd read anyway and I hoped it was true. Especially now that I was pregnant, I worried about being exposed to too many diseases.

I grabbed a new patient chart out of a desk drawer

and walked over to the counter to get the glass thermometer and portable blood pressure machine to take Lee's vital signs. I glanced out the window at the snow. Through the hanging kudzu vines, bare now except for a few shriveled browned leaves, I could see cars moving slowly in the gray slush along Belvidere Street.

"Wow. It's really coming down now. You got a place to stay tonight?" I asked.

I listened for Lee's answer and was reassured that he had a bed in the Bunkhouse shelter downstairs. The social workers mainly kept these beds for men who were sick—a sort of medical respite facility. It was snowing hard enough that I wondered if I would have to leave my car in the back parking lot of the Street Center and walk north on Belvidere the two or so miles home. The idea of the walk didn't bother me, since I was still running several miles a day and was in good physical shape. But I'd have to leave well before dark. The two-mile walk home would take me through Jackson Ward, an impoverished and stereotyped "crime-ridden" black neighborhood. I lived on the other side of Jackson Ward, in the mostly white middle-class Ginter Park neighborhood, near the Presbyterian seminary where my husband was a student.

Lee didn't have a fever and his lungs sounded only slightly congested, so I gave him a small bottle of cough syrup and did a tuberculosis test on him, placing the medicine under the skin of his forearm with a small needle. I instructed him to come back to see me in two days so I could read the test results. He told me he had been working several years as a janitor in the plasma center downtown, but had recently been fired, so he was working in day-labor pools sweeping up at construction sites. He was too slightly built to look capable of doing heavy construction or garden work, the main types of day-labor work available in Richmond. I finished up with him and left work early to drive home.

Lee came back to see me two days later, saying he still had a cough but was feeling better and was able to work. I checked his arm and his tuberculosis test was negative. Then Lee disappeared from the Street Center for five months. When he returned he was noticeably thinner. He told me he was coughing up blood and waking up at night drenched in sweat—classic signs of tuberculosis. So I retested him for tuberculosis and drew blood for HIV and syphilis, just to be sure. His only risk factor for HIV seemed to be his work at the plasma center; he told me he'd had more than a few puncture wounds from used needles lying around as he was cleaning up. I knew that someone with AIDS could have tuberculosis and not show it on an initial skin test. From the marked change in Lee's appearance, I had a bad feeling about what the test results would show. Richmond-area doctors were just beginning to see an increasing number of patients with full-blown AIDS, and most patients were being referred to infectious disease specialists at the Medical College of Virginia—MCV—hospital, Richmond's state-run academic medical center.

My bad feeling was confirmed. Lee was diagnosed with advanced AIDS and disseminated tuberculosis—tuberculosis that was not only in his lungs, but also in his spinal cord and bone marrow. I helped hold him still in MCV hospital when doctors drilled a large needle into his hip bone for a sample of marrow to confirm the diagnosis. It's the only time I ever saw Lee cry.

For several months he lived in the Street Center's Bunkhouse shelter downstairs, and spent his days with me upstairs in the newly expanded clinic. By then the clinic had moved down the hall into a new addition built on the back of the

Street Center. I now had two exam rooms with exam tables, a bathroom, a small waiting room, and a dental clinic with a dental chair used only on Saturdays. To save money in the construction, the new clinic had only one small vertical window, located in my office beside my desk. The window didn't open. It looked out over the Street Center's back parking lot. Even though the new clinic space was more functional than what I had started off with, the lack of natural light and a window that opened made me miss my old office.

I gave Lee his daily tuberculosis medication injection, trying to find remaining thigh muscle to plunge the two-inch needle into. The medication I had to inject was bright white and thick, the consistency of wet concrete. I dreaded giving him the shots; it seemed like torture as I squeezed it slowly into his flesh. Lee never complained. After the shot, he'd swallow his other medications, curl up in the empty orange plastic dental chair, turn on the overhead exam lamp, and do crossword puzzles between naps. I'd throw an old Army blanket over his shriveled form. Toward the end of the clinic day, he'd emerge from the dental room, roll himself around the waiting room on an exam stool, laugh, and greet people in his affable, goofy way. Lee knew how to make me laugh; he appointed himself the clinic jester. He told me not to take things so seriously.

I was taking things seriously. I was a new mother, working full-time to support my family while my husband finished seminary. At the Street Center Clinic I was seeing an increasing number of homeless patients with complex social and health problems, and I was still the only health care provider. I was having a hard time keeping up with everything in my life.

While I had to give Lee daily injections, I was terrified of becoming infected with HIV from a contaminated needle. I tried not to wear gloves when I was working with Lee; I knew he already felt like an outcast, a leper, an untouchable. But when I gave him shots I wore two pairs of gloves. By then we mostly knew how the HIV virus was spread, but we had no medicine to prevent it in case of an accidental needle stick. Soon after I returned to clinic from maternity leave in May, I was forced to temporarily stop nursing my son when I had a needle stick, until I confirmed the patient was HIV and hepatitis negative. I still wasn't sure how far I'd go, what I'd risk catching in the name of compassion, of health care duty.

———————

Not long after I finished the month-long series of injections and Lee was taking medications on his own, I got a phone call.

"Nurse Jo, you got to come get me out of this place. Talk to them and tell them I'm not crazy!"

The police had picked up Lee in nearby Monroe Park, because he was talking loudly to himself and dancing around barefoot on frozen grass in November. Monroe Park was a block-wide city park just north of the Street Center. The park was surrounded by the campus of the state college, Virginia Commonwealth University (VCU). MCV hospital, where Lee usually went for specialty care for his tuberculosis and AIDS, was the medical campus of VCU. MCV hospital was located in the downtown business core, next door to the White House of the Confederacy, and a half-mile east of Monroe Park. A Victorian-era park with gnarled old magnolia and oak trees, cast-iron benches, and a central fountain, Monroe Park was a popular hangout for college students, as well as for homeless people. It was especially popular with homeless people like Lee.

"Where are you? Have you been taking your pills?" I grabbed a pen and some scrap paper, and then pulled his medical chart out of a file cabinet, quickly scanning his medication list that had grown to several pages in length.

Lee hadn't been taking the medication that kept the swelling around his brain from causing hallucinations. The police had escorted him to a small private hospital up the street from the Street Center. I wasn't sure why the police had taken him there instead of to MCV. Perhaps it was because the private hospital was closer and more convenient for them. MCV hospital had Lee's medical records, and doctors there could have figured out what was wrong with him more quickly. Lee was calling me from the locked psychiatric ward of the private hospital where he was being held for observation. The doctors had involuntarily committed him to an inpatient psychiatric unit because they considered him a threat to himself or to others; I wasn't sure which, since he'd been in Monroe Park acting crazy and probably scaring students. Legally, they could hold him forty-eight hours for observation, but he had to have a hearing on the second day with a court magistrate who would decide whether or not to release him.

The next morning I showed up at the hospital to testify at his hearing. In the hospital lobby, I had to take a special elevator that only stopped on the seventh-floor psychiatric unit. There was a secret code to make this elevator work. It always seems like people look at you funny when you ask to take the psychiatric-floor elevator; even being around crazy people is stigmatizing. Once on the floor, I had to show my ID, sign in, and be escorted onto the unit by a burly bouncer of a male nurse. The entry was through a heavy metal door. As it closed with a thud behind me, I could feel the air sucked out of the hallway I had stepped into. I had a vision of Nurse Ratched in *One Flew Over the Cuckoo's Nest*; she was locking me inside. I swallowed my panic.

We walked down an empty corridor painted that peculiarly putrid shade of hospital green, and entered a sunny, overly warm conference room. Sitting around the rectangular table were four middle-aged white men, two in dark suits and ties, and two in white coats. The white coats were, of course, Lee's doctors, and the others were the court magistrate and his assistant. It was a corner room with ceiling-to-floor windows on two sides, the sun streaming in on the men clustered at that end. I had to squint into the sun to look at them while I decided where I should sit.

"Nurse Jo, thanks for coming!" Lee was huddled in a chair close to the door.

"Of course I would come." I brushed his shoulder with my hand as I sat down beside him.

Lee was dressed in several layers of blue hospital gowns, with the vulnerable air that clings to them. When the magistrate began his questioning, Lee kept his head down, answering just yes or no in a barely audible whisper. The hearing went quickly. At the end, the magistrate decided to release Lee, with the provision that he continue taking his medications under my supervision. I had to sign a form acknowledging responsibility for Lee's care. Otherwise, the magistrate said, Lee was a public health threat. Lee came back to the Street Center that afternoon carrying a white plastic hospital bag full of blue stretchy hospital slippers, a toothbrush, and pages of typed-up discharge instructions.

Soon after the hospital stay, Lee grew more tired and wanted a place of his own. The Street Center social worker helped him find a low-rent room. It was in a house near the clinic, in a decaying section of the traditionally all-black neighborhood of Jackson Ward, around the corner from a life-sized bronze Bojangles dancing on stairs. Bojangles had been born and raised in Jackson Ward. Lee came back to the Street Center every day in the outreach van for a hot meal and medications. The van driver told me he had to throw pebbles at the second-floor front window where Lee lived to let him know he was there; the house had no doorbell. The driver had never been inside the house and neither had the social worker.

Lee didn't answer the van driver's pebbles three days in a row and the social worker was on vacation, so I decided to check on Lee. It was a cold, bright day in mid-December. I pulled up in my car at the address given to me by the van driver. There was a block of row houses, most with boarded-up windows, and several in black-charred ruins. The sidewalk, street, and houses were all deserted: no people, no stray dogs or cats, not even a squirrel. The emptiness and stark sunlight and shadows were evocative of an Edward Hopper painting, with the haunting beauty of loneliness.

No one answered the door when I knocked, so I looked for pebbles to throw at the window, wondering which size wouldn't break the glass. The small square patch of dirt at the base of the front steps was bare except for a frozen pile of dog excrement. I walked to a pot-holed area of the street and found pieces of gravel, wondering if I could get arrested for vandalism, hoping the police wouldn't cruise by.

Still not getting any response after throwing the gravel at his window, I walked down to the street corner where the landlord's office was located. A plump black woman sat behind a desk marked Property Manager. I explained who I was and that I needed to check on Lee as I was concerned about his health. "Oh that Lee! He's probably just coming down off a drunk," she said in response. That surprised me. I knew Lee had been a drinker in the past, but I hadn't noticed or heard of any evidence of it in the past six months. I thought Lee was too sick to drink. But I figured it wasn't worth challenging her judgment. She sighed heavily while pushing herself up from the chair, then cuffed a large metal ring of keys hanging on the wall.

"Come on, let's go see."

I followed her down the street. She walked fast, swaying side to side, and breathing heavily, sending out clouds of condensation into the cold air around her.

After she opened the front door of Lee's building to reveal a dark hallway, she didn't try to turn on the lights: the building had no electricity. There was enough sunlight from the curtainless windows to reveal the side rooms, empty except for floors strewn with paper bags from fast-food places, empty beer cans, and liquor bottles. There seemed to be no one in the house. As I followed the woman up the stairs, a piece of wooden railing fell off under my hand. It clattered to the floor below, raising a puff of dust. I was worried I'd broken something of her property, but she didn't seem to notice. I continued to climb the stairs, now worried that I might fall through myself. Then a smell began to reach me, a smell I struggled to identify, then remembered: it was the sweet-sick smell of human decay, of putrid flesh.

I turned to the left at the top of the stairs, walked past an overflowing toilet reeking of human excrement—there was no running water either—and past a room occupied by a half-burned mattress on the floor. Still there were no people. The property manager was breezy, businesslike; she did not seem to see or smell or be concerned about anything in the house. I'd been under bridges and in homeless encampments on river mudflats that were more fit for human habitation. I wondered how someone could live here, how someone could charge money for someone to live here. Weren't there laws against this kind of thing?

At a closed door in the front of the house, she rattled the key ring. "Lee, you in there?" She didn't knock but began to fling the door open.

"Yeah. I'm here," we heard faintly from inside.

"Okay. The nurse is here to see you." She turned to me, "I gotta get back to the office." As she walked away she bellowed over her shoulder, "Now behave yourself Lee! You hear me?" She didn't wait for his answer as she disappeared down the stairs.

Lee was sitting hunched over on a folding cot inside the door. The room was not a room, but rather a walk-in closet with a small window. The cot, a paper bag, and a small kerosene heater were all that fit in the space. Lee looked up at me with his dark eyes. His face was ashen. Between his feet on the floor was a yellow hospital basin half filled with frothy pale-pink spit. Lee's breathing was so fast and shallow he could barely speak.

"I wondered . . . when . . . you'd get here," he panted, grinning up at me.

"Lee, you look like hell. When did it get this bad?" I stalled for time, half listening to his answer, thinking I'd have to call an ambulance, thinking I'd have to go back down to the property manager's office to borrow her phone to call an ambulance, thinking I didn't want to see her again. I couldn't understand how black people could prey upon other black people, followed by the awkward realization that this assumption was naive and racist. But still, I didn't want to see her again, and felt indignant that she was part of a system that allowed people to live like this.

Lee refused an ambulance, complaining of mounting medical bills he couldn't pay. I didn't point out that he wasn't going to live long enough for the bills to matter—that seemed cruel. He agreed to let me take him to MCV hospital in my car. He was skinny enough by then that I could half carry him down the stairs and out to my car.

This went against everything I had been taught in nursing school about appropriate professional boundaries with patients. As I tucked Lee into the front seat of my car, the stern countenances of several nursing instructors flashed in my memory, along with their maxims: "Never transport a patient in your own car! Do not get overly invested emotionally with a patient! Stop when you think you may be going too far!"

I ignored their voices, and whisked Lee down the street to the hospital and then into the emergency department in a wheelchair, insisting he be seen right away, saying he was in respiratory distress, using medical code words and knowing I was being labeled a troublemaker by the jaded staff. I was wearing jeans, a sweater, and a coat, but no lab coat or nametag to identify myself as a health care professional. I knew how hospitals worked, especially this hospital, since it was where I had gone to nursing school. They let us bypass the waiting room and Lee got admitted to a medical unit.

Getting too close to my patients was something I was taught not to do. Health care providers are supposed to maintain a healthy emotional distance. A distance to prevent being so overwhelmed by emotions that it cripples the provision of proper health care. A distance to prevent professional burnout. It sounds good in theory, but there's no way to teach someone where that boundary is, or to know where it is for yourself. The business of nursing brings us into the messy swampland of human suffering, illness, and death. It is impossible to erect walls or channel rivers within a swamp. So, healthy emotional distance, what is it in such terrain?

When I visited Lee the next day, his nurse asked me to help him fill out consent forms for what he wanted when he couldn't breathe on his own: did he want only comfort measures or to be put on a breathing machine? He was alone in an isolation room because they weren't sure if he had another contagious disease. I had to don a fluttering canary-yellow paper gown, vinyl gloves, and a paper mask before I went into his room. It seemed silly since I'd already been exposed to whatever he might have, but Lee's nurse put her hands on her hips and glared at me until I put on all the items. Then she handed me the forms and walked back to the nurses' station. I stared at her retreating form. There's something about the rigid rules of hospitals that brings out my rebellious streak. I knew I would never last long working in a hospital. That's why I had chosen community health where I had more freedom—and more complications—I mused as I opened the door to Lee's room.

Lee was lying in bed, an IV dripping through a needle and tubing into his right arm, a steamy plastic oxygen mask whooshing over his face. He woke up, nodded, and smiled when I walked in. I pulled off my mask and said hello.

The consent form was one page, front and back, with Lee's patient labels affixed to the top. The form was on a brown clipboard that had a ballpoint pen attached to the clip by a string. I took off my gloves, pulled out the form, and quickly scanned it. I had read these forms before in patient charts, but had never helped a patient complete them; family members or the patient's doctor always did this.

"Lee, they want me to help you with this form about your medical care choices. You want me to read it to you?"

He nodded, so I read it out loud, stopping occasionally to explain a medical term or procedure to him, but trying not to express my own opinions of the options mentioned on the form by way of either words or facial expressions. By then, Lee knew he probably wasn't leaving the hospital. He told me he was tired of being ill and so he signed the Do Not Resuscitate form. I wasn't sure if I had been neutral enough in explaining it to him. I didn't want him to suffer. I knew there were worse things than death. After he signed the forms he told me he wanted a chocolate milkshake from his favorite fast-food place. He smiled through his oxygen mask when he said this.

I had to finish some work at the clinic, and when I returned with the milkshake, Lee was in the intensive care unit, hooked up to a breathing machine. His nurse told me that when Lee's breathing worsened to the point he couldn't talk, he had nodded yes to having changed his mind about the consent forms. I was dubious, but then, I hadn't been there. And I didn't know how it felt to slowly suffocate. It did cross my mind that this was a teaching hospital, and that perhaps doctors wanted to prolong Lee's life as teaching fodder for young physicians. I pushed these thoughts away.

Lee quickly went into a coma, spiking a temperature of close to 110°F, higher than I'd known was possible. They placed Lee's bloated but emaciated body on a bed-sized blue ice pad over an air mattress that noisily sucked in and out along with the softer sighs of his breathing machine. Wrapped in white sheets and lying on a raftlike bed, it was as if Lee was being ferried by Charon to the underworld.

He lingered in that state for days, then over a week. Finally, his medical team called for an ethics committee meeting to decide whether or not to remove him from all the machines keeping him alive, lingering, here and not here. They asked me to be at the meeting. I found myself in another hospital conference room with his doctors and the hospital chaplain. The Street Center social worker had been trying to find Lee's family members ever since he was first hospitalized. No family members had been located. I sat at one end of the conference table. Lee's senior doctor was droning on, reciting dry medical facts about Lee's case in a precise, organized manner, looking up from his notes to the ceiling and back down again, as if lost in a soliloquy.

The doctors discussed Lee's case for a half hour, at the end of which his medical team voted to stop the machines the next day. I was relieved they didn't ask me to vote, but they did ask me what I thought Lee would have wanted. I told them he was tired of being ill, and that if he couldn't get better, he wanted to die.

After the meeting, I went back to Lee's bed, behind the white curtain separating him from other critically ill patients. He was alone in his curtained space. I touched his burning hand and said a silent good-bye.

I stood at the end of his bed contemplating what else to do, wondering what was proper. Do you just say good-bye and leave, or do you say something more profound, make solemn, grand promises like "Lee, I will make sure no one ever dies like this again"—and isn't that just a bit too grand and narcissistic? But that is what I said.

Not wanting to leave too hastily, I glanced down and saw his aluminum-clad medical chart hanging from a rack at the end of his bed. Now curious what the hospital knew about Lee that I didn't, I grabbed the chart and quickly scanned through it from the back forwards: results of numerous blood tests, recordings of Lee's vital signs, and pages of flowery handwritten nurses' notes with entries such as "patient resting comfortably." On the first page of the chart on a typed intake form, I noticed my name beside the category "Next of Kin." My first reaction was shock that the hospital staff had made such a mistake: how could a young Nordic-looking white girl like me be this black man's next of kin? I closed the chart and hung it back in its rack before the nurses could come in and scold me for reading through it.

Now I knew: I'd gotten too close to this patient of mine. Lee and I were bound by something like blood. And I had yet another tie to this complex land of the South—a land that both fascinated and repulsed me.

CHAPTER TWO

First Families

I GREW UP TEN miles northeast of Oakwood Cemetery where Lee now lies buried. I was raised on a six-hundred-acre Christian camp surrounded by Civil War ghosts. I was the only real Virginian in my family. My father's family was from Georgia and Tennessee, lawyers, judges, and cotton farmers. My mother was Pennsylvania Dutch, completely from the North. My three older siblings had been born in North Carolina many years before I was born.

The dirt road to my house was built on the remains of the corduroy road made by the Union Army a century before I was born. My mother told me it was called corduroy because the Army cut trunks of Virginia red cedar and laid the logs crosswise on the road through marshy areas to keep their cannons from getting stuck. There was a section of the corduroy road that cut through the woods where our road ended and a footpath continued. The logs were still there in places, dark, slippery with muck and black swirly rainbow-slicked water, sucking in and out as I walked over them, releasing rotten gassy smells.

The land I grew up on near Cold Harbor had been the site of the bloodiest battles in the Civil War. The two battles were two years apart; soldiers on both sides in the last battle unearthed decomposing bodies from the previous battle as they dug trenches. Our land was strewn with Civil War bullets, musket balls, deep earthworks, and mounded graves. Long before, the Pamunkey Indians had scattered the land with white quartz arrowheads. My mother collected arrowheads and bullets along the road. When I was a child, she taught me how to search for them.

———————

There was a path behind our house that began at the swing set, wandered through holly bushes, gangly sassafras, and towering oak trees draped in honeysuckle, passionflower, and poison ivy vines, then connected with the pot-holed dirt road leading out of camp. Before I was old enough to start school, this was the path my mother and I walked after lunch to get the mail. We searched for bullets along the way. Spring was my favorite time to go for walks. The wild dogwoods spattered the woods with white flowered snow in amongst the new green shoots of leaves shimmering in the sun. Sometimes my mother found flat metal buttons from soldiers' jackets. Other times she found old bullets with smashed-in points.

"These are ones that hit something and got smashed," my mother said, holding up a buff-colored bullet for me to see.

"Hit something like what?" I asked, gazing up at her.

"Well, like maybe trees or people. It hit their bones and that's what killed them." She'd tell me things like this even though I was only four and had a hard time sleeping. At night, I'd lie awake thinking of bullets.

On these springtime walks I pretended to look for arrowheads and bullets, but what I really searched for were violets. Wood violets were shy flowers, growing under the shade of young sassafras trees and cinnamon ferns, between the mossy cedar logs of the corduroy road. I loved their heart-shaped leaves, deep purple or purple-veined white flowers, and honeyed scent. The purple-veined violets were less common and were called Confederate violets, because from a distance their color resembled the faded blue-gray of Confederate uniforms.

I saw my first ghost on a spring day. I was walking on the path to the mailbox with my mother. She was up ahead, stooped over with her hands clasped behind her back, walking slowly, while gently swaying from side to side searching for bullets. I lagged behind looking for violets and found a large patch beside a white oak tree. I knelt down to smell the violets, inhaling their aching sweetness, a scent that in the next moment became the combined essence of fear and enchantment. Beside the violets I saw a half-buried bullet. As if it were one of my marbles, I flicked the bullet with an index finger, and saw it had a smashed tip. In a flash, I saw the bone and the crumpled body of the soldier the bullet had entered. I froze, feeling warmth slowly thaw my neck, hearing echoes of my heartbeat deep inside my head. Before I knew what I was doing, I buried the bullet down in the spongy earth and covered it with a mound of violets. My heart still bounding, I ran to catch up with my mother. I didn't tell her what I had seen and she never asked why I stopped looking for bullets.

I saw other ghosts on our land, where they tended cows, farmed tobacco and corn, and fetched water from streams. They didn't bother me the way the ghost of the soldier had, but I didn't tell my mother about these either. I collected sights of them along with other secrets of my childhood, secrets that over time hardened into the skeleton of my identity. The ghosts lived near old fallen-down houses on the other side of the lake, along vestiges of the old corduroy road. I'd see them out of the corner of my eye as I walked amongst the silver lichen-clad pine trees growing straight in the rounded fur- rows of the overgrown farm fields. Sometimes they glowed at night in the foxfire fungi and swamp gas in marshy areas surrounding my house.

On our property there were three of these houses aban- doned after the Civil War, now flattened jumbles of wood covered by Virginia creeper. Old daffodils bloomed around the houses in spring, and magenta climbing roses gasped through thick mildewed leaves in June. Each house had a deep open well nearby, full of tree limbs and snakes, fenced off because people had fallen in them and had to be res- cued before they got bitten by copperheads and died down there. That's what my mother told me, holding my hand as I gazed over the edge into the dark pit. I was fascinated and repulsed, full of an alchemy of agony and awe. Secretly I wanted to crawl inside those grottoes and touch their drip- ping moss-covered sides.

My mother took me on expeditions to these houses. First, she would study a large blown-up aerial photograph of the camp property. She'd point to an area of the map: "See those patches of dark green? That's where an old house used to be. The green is from all the old walnut trees they planted around it." Then, armed with bags and garden trowels, we'd set off on trails through the woods. Once we'd found a house site, she'd locate the refuse area nearby and we would start digging, finding pale-turquoise baking soda bottles, leather boots, enameled rusted-through buckets, and iron spokes from wagon wheels. In eroded red-and-gray clay banks of streams near the houses, we found fossil seashells and sharks' teeth. At four, I understood the history of our land in a jumbled Alice in Wonderland sort of way, imagining Indians and Civil War soldiers fighting undersea sharks.

The ghosts of the people who had lived around the old houses seemed content. Near one of the houses was a family burial site. Leaf-strewn mounds of earth bumped together in a line like the cedar logs on the corduroy road. The site was on a bluff overlooking a ravine cascading down to a small stream. Most of the graves had carved gray headstones: Robert Anderson born March 10, 1792, died July 26, 1853; William Nelson Anderson born February 16, 1837, died May 15, 1851; and, Nancy Peasley Anderson born April 18, 1833, died July 15, 1834. Nancy's grave was short, but there was an even-shorter grave next to it of another Nancy, "infant granddaughter" Nancy Julia Elizabeth with no dates given. A few feet away were six or so bigger unmarked graves, which my mother said were those of Negro slaves. These couldn't have been content, but I didn't see their ghosts back then. It was as if they had never existed. The idea of Negro slaves was something I vaguely understood. I knew that slavery was a Southern sin, something to be regretted, something to move away from.

I absorbed history from our land before being taught proper Virginia history in grade school. Once I began school at Battlefield Park Elementary School, my textbooks had pastel-colored drawings depicting the Godspeed, Susan Constant, and the Discovery tall ships of Jamestown, and another of Pocahontas, looking like a Barbie Doll in a bikini. The boys in my class twittered over this page. There was an illustration of thick-lipped black slaves on a Richmond auction block, but I don't remember any discussion of slavery or race relations in school. Strange, since around us roiled the Civil Rights Movement, my school was desegregated when I was in second grade, and in the spring of that year Martin Luther King, Jr. was assassinated. What I remember about the year of desegregation is that my school bus began picking up black kids along our route. They sat together in the back of the bus. When I asked my mother about this, she said it was out of habit, and that they probably felt better sitting together.

The only history I was taught in school, until grade eight at Stonewall Jackson Junior High School, was Virginia history, as if there were no worlds outside the Commonwealth. At night, when I was reading my history textbook, my mother would frown over my shoulder, scan the page, make guttural "Hmmm" sounds, and mutter, "Well, that's not exactly correct." I'd look up from my book and she would provide me with an alternative view of Virginia history, such as, "The early English settlers here were prisoners and women who got into trouble and got kicked out of England. Remember that when anyone tells you they're Virginia Blueblood or from Virginia's so-called First Families."

My mother was an educated woman, a professional artist. She had a master's degree in fine arts from a university in the North. I figured she knew more about most things than did my provincial teachers and textbooks. Not surprisingly, in fourth grade when history was graded separately, I didn't do well. On the back of my report card, my mother wrote in beautiful cursive, "I have felt for some time that I should talk with Mrs. Blaylock about her social studies tests and the history textbook used. Please let me know when would be a convenient time."

I do wonder how that conversation went between my mother and my fourth-grade teacher. I never asked. As I have come to know now, this was during an era of the Virginia Blueblood oligarchy control of school textbooks. Liberal, educated voters like my parents were fighting this control. Members of the First Families of Virginia, such as the Byrds, Carters, Lees, and Berkeleys, controlled the State legislature and decided the appropriate version of Virginia history that could be taught. Our school field trips seemed approved by them as well, and were to places like the White House of the Confederacy, Monticello, and the Shirley and Tuckahoe Plantations—all former or current homes of the First Families. I did not go to school with children of Virginia Bluebloods. The white children I was in school with were children of farmers or small tradesmen who lived in LEGO-shaped ranch houses with incongruous pillared antebellum flourishes, black lawn jockeys, and stone deer in their front yards.

The camp I grew up in was opened in 1957 as the first racially integrated children's summer camp in the South. It was Presbyterian, but also ecumenical and interfaith. My father was recruited from his North Carolina church to open it. My father was a tempestuous man with an unpredictable, explosive temper. It probably required a difficult person like my father to challenge the deeply ingrained racism of the South by opening a racially integrated camp on the outskirts of the capital of the Confederacy.

Handsome, athletically built on an average frame, with piercing blue eyes, a firm square jaw, and a wide grin, my father was relentlessly gregarious. He greeted strangers with a firm handshake and friendly banter. People said he was delightful, and he was—at times. My father was an excellent storyteller; he had a strong voice and a dramatic, charismatic presence. He was a natural entertainer, using animated hand movements when he talked. My father was in the circus as a boy and he could still walk on his hands up flights of stairs when I was a child. He created a mesmerizing force field around himself that dictated what could and could not be talked about in his presence—that dictated what was real and unreal.

The summer camp had racially integrated staff and campers. Summers were full of canoe trips on the nearby rivers, volleyball games in the dust, sliding like otters on wet clay hillsides beside the lake, cookouts, and campfires. My father presided over each solemn opening and closing campfire deep in the nighttime woods, reciting the poem, "Kneel always when you light a fire! Kneel reverently and thankful be" as he lit the fire, a circle of restless faces gathered around. The faces of white children glowed in the firelight, while the black faces stayed hidden.

Most of the black kids who came to camp were "welfare kids" or "charity kids" because they were from the poor inner-city housing projects, like those in Jackson Ward. I felt sorry for the black kids. My parents encouraged me to love them out of Christian duty.

If there were local tensions about our camp being integrated, I wasn't aware of them. I lived for my summers and got through the school year by washing dishes for diverse weekend retreat groups at camp, such as the B'nai B'rith Jewish Youth and Southern Baptist missionary kids. There was even a large Hindu meditation group led by a wizened, straggly gray-haired Indian on a hot-pink plastic lounge chair surrounded by flaming marigolds. Camp expanded my world past Virginia, past the South, past the Civil War ghosts that continued to swirl around and through me. No longer frightening, the ghosts had become part of the landscape.

———————

One late summer day I was riding in our VW bug. My mother was driving on back roads from the airport, within view of downtown Richmond, not far from Oakwood Cemetery. We had just dropped off a camp counselor who was flying back to college. I was ten, sitting in the backseat, slumped against the right side window, reading a book, vaguely registering the countryside and farms we were passing, when my mother slammed on the brakes.

"Damn!" I never heard my mother curse, so I looked up quickly.

"What?" I asked.

"Keep your head down and stay quiet," she said, adding more softly as she turned off the engine, "It'll be okay." I could see her leaning forwards, both hands tightly clutching the top of the steering wheel. I slumped down in the seat while quickly peering out the side window to see what had stopped us, to see what would be okay, to see what she didn't want me to see. I figured it was a bad car accident and she didn't want me to see the dead or injured people.

It was approaching dusk, the witching magic hour for the waning sun. The field next to us glowed golden, with large rectangular hay bales strewn about the field of wheat-stalk stubble. Hovering over the field, suspended in the thick damp evening air, were shining motes of hay bits, effervescent like Fourth of July sparklers. With our car engine turned off, the sound of cicadas and crickets created a curtain of white noise, as mesmerizing as the floating hay.

"Evening, ma'am. Don't mean no trouble. I gotta stop

you here awhile. There's a meeting that's passing through, that's all. You can get going in a minute or so." I heard the man's voice, polite, official-sounding, with crisp words stuck in a slow Southern drawl, as it came in my mother's open window. I looked between the seats and saw a spotless white-gloved hand cupped over the doorsill. Behind that was blazing white with a thin, trickling, blood-red cross, and above the cross was no face within a white mask, pale thin lips moving within an elliptical cutout area. From the words spoken and the weight of the voice, I expected to see the uniform of a policeman. When I first saw the white mask, I felt disoriented and had to remind myself it wasn't Halloween. I stayed quiet, huddled down behind the seats. As the man walked away, I looked out the front windshield to see where he was going. Up ahead, perhaps fifty feet away, was a swarm of ghostly pointed-hat masked figures swirling around a huge bonfire. It took a moment for me to see that inside the bonfire was a ten-foot dark wooden cross.

"What's that and why are they wearing those weird costumes?" I asked.

"Shhhhh—I'll tell you later. Stay down and stay quiet," my mother said.

Absorbing the fear in my mother's voice, I sank deeper in the seat, but moved over to the middle so I could see out the front windshield at the fire and the figures. Several of the white-clad men reached into the fire with long wooden sticks and withdrew flaming torches. Then en masse, with fluid amoeboid movement, the group came toward us, sucking in lone figures as it streamed forward. I heard deep-voiced chanting, words indecipherable as a foreign language. They grew louder, surrounding our car, lighting the inside with their glowing whiteness and lit torches, gently rocking the car as they brushed past it, moving across the road, then thinning to double-file down a dirt path that cut through the next field. The comforting, familiar smell of wood smoke followed them.

I didn't hear my mother start the car. We were speeding away, screeching around bends in the road. Reflected in the rearview mirror, I saw my mother's face set hard as stone, etched with the fierce anger I seldom saw. I was more afraid of her anger than I had been of the men we had seen. I stayed quiet, huddled down in the backseat, bracing myself for the rough ride. When we got home, she disappeared into her bedroom, talking quietly with my father—so quietly that I couldn't make out what they were saying, even with my ear pressed against the rough stucco wall between our bedrooms.

At the dinner table that night, my father told me we had been in the middle of a Ku Klux Klan meeting. "They're racist white men who wear those costumes to look like ghosts of Confederate soldiers to scare black people, and to scare white people who don't agree with them, like it scared your mother." As I slowly chewed a mouthful of food, I considered this information. The ghostly man who had stopped us seemed polite, a Southern gentleman. Being in the midst of the KKK meeting had been exotic, dreamlike, seductive—almost beautiful. I knew that what I had seen, the way I had seen it, was not something to discuss. I swallowed the dissonance between my mother's reaction and my own experience of the encounter.

The dissonance remains. It took living out of and looking back at the South to understand that ghosts becoming part of the landscape are not something to relax into. The landscape of my childhood is a landscape of half-buried violence, covered with violets, punctuated by deep, abandoned wells. The roads leading back to it are as twisted as the country roads I grew up on. Within the accretive layers of nostalgia lies the sludge of orange dust, tasting of blood. I both fear and yearn for the complexity, the offbeat rhythm of the South that has formed me.

CHAPTER THREE

Foreign Territory

IN EARLY MAY 1986 I opened the CrossOver Clinic at the Richmond Street Center. I was twenty-five years old and completing graduate nursing school. I'd talked my way into this job as the sole health care provider at the newly opened Street Center. This was the middle of the Reagan years, with the ascendancy of the Moral Majority. On the horizon was the glimmer of soon-to-be President Bush and his Thousand Points of Light. I saw myself as one of those points of light, young and passionate about my work with the burgeoning number of homeless people living on our city streets. This was why, on my first official day of clinic, I had a needle in my arm. I was passionate and had no idea what I was doing. The HIV/AIDS epidemic was just beginning, and accompanying it came the return of tuberculosis. Knowing I'd have to be doing a lot of screening for tuberculosis, I decided to do a skin test, practicing on my own arm.

Over the past few weeks I had painted the walls and stocked the shelves of the clinic. The clinic consisted of one newly whitewashed corner office on the third floor of the flat-roofed redbrick warehouse at the corner of Canal and Belvidere Streets. On this first day of clinic, I sat at a battered yellow enameled metal desk, my straight blonde hair pulled back severely in an Amish-girl sort of ponytail. I wore no makeup, a shin-length navy skirt, and a white shirt, fully buttoned. An old-fashioned black leather doctor's bag sat on the desk in front of me. I looked younger than I was and I knew it. I had a difficult time being taken seriously as a nurse because of it, so I tried to dress matronly and carried a white lab coat in case I needed the extra air of authority.

My medical equipment included a portable blood pressure machine from the 1950s, a cheap neon-green plastic stethoscope, mercury-filled glass thermometers, and a six-inch microscope from a child's science set. One of the volunteer doctors who did medical missions' work in impoverished countries had donated the toy microscope. When he first brought it to the clinic as we were setting up, I thought it was a joke, until he explained he used it in Haiti because it was portable and didn't require electricity. We viewed this clinic as a medical mission akin to those in developing countries. The homeless were exotic, impoverished, foreign-to-us people.

I sat behind my desk, bare left forearm extended with my right hand-holding the needle horizontally in my arm. Then I looked up and saw a man gazing placidly at me from the doorway.

"May I help you?" I asked, holding the needle steady.

He didn't answer. He was ebony-skinned, bone-thin,

short, and dreadlocked. He wore faded jeans shredded at the ankles, duct tape for a belt, an old half-buttoned flannel shirt, and a floppy Rastafarian multicolored beret perched on his matted hair. He had a backpack slung over one shoulder, and he was eating a donut. There were gooey crumbs and white powdered sugar all over his scraggly beard.

The image of a freshly scrubbed young white girl with a needle in her arm didn't seem to faze him. It did faze me. How do you begin to explain having a needle in your arm to a person you don't know? I was eager to make a good impression, establish trust and rapport with the clients and staff of the Street Center, and I realized this wasn't going to help. From the way he looked, I figured the man standing in my doorway wasn't a staff member.

Louie was a consumer, as the social workers at the Street Center referred to the people who came there for services. And he was soon to be my first patient. No one at the Street Center knew Louie's last name; Louie didn't seem to know himself, or was too paranoid to tell us. He claimed he was in his late twenties and had lived in Richmond all his life. He had severe paranoid schizophrenia and was covered with head and body lice. He lived behind the green metal dumpster in the Street Center parking lot, making a shelter for himself out of old discarded wooden doors and orange vinyl couches, with a cardboard handwritten sign over the entrance proclaiming: "Keep Out. My home." He mumbled constantly to himself, but rarely talked. The day he walked into clinic he didn't say a word. He just looked at me while he slowly chewed his donut, and then he wandered off.

As I finished my tuberculosis test and busied myself in the empty clinic, I tried to quiet my rising panic. I had barely met the staff of the two lead agencies in the building, and I didn't know if I'd fit in. What would the patients be like? Would I even have any patients? If I did have patients, would I be able to provide the right health care for them, or would I accidentally kill them? On top of that, I was creating my job as I went along. I was a novice nurse working alone in the clinic during the week. It was all uncharted terrain. And now I wondered if the man with the donut was running downstairs to tell people the new nurse was shooting up in the clinic. I hurriedly put all the packages of needles away in a drawer in case someone else came in.

I stared at the small black plastic microscope sitting on the window ledge. I thought about my childhood dreams of becoming a great scientist or missionary doctor, going off to exotic countries to cure the world of hunger and disease. Albert Schweitzer was big back then, as was developing a protein-enriched rice strain to keep people from starving. My family was riddled with Christian zealots, ministers, and missionaries—my father and grandfather, uncles—I'd lost count of them all. As a teenager, I wanted nothing more than to get out of the ghost-filled woods of Virginia, to go to college up North, then perhaps to Africa or some other exotic place, and never come back. Restless, seeking adventure, I had gone to a mostly Midwestern college (Oberlin) and to a decidedly Northern university seminary (Harvard). Now I was back in the South, and it was feeling like foreign territory.

Three years before I opened the Street Center Clinic I moved back to Richmond from Boston to go to nursing school. The first year of nursing school I lived in a dorm room near the main MCV hospital located on Shockoe Hill. Shockoe

Hill was in a dismal corner of the city, sandwiched between two interstates, a train yard, low-income housing projects, and the decaying Jackson Ward. To the south of the hospital, across Broad Street, were the State Capitol, state legislative buildings, and the James River. My dorm room was on the ninth floor with a window overlooking the city jail.

Nursing school classes were simplistic and boring. I did a private reading on fetal brain development with a medical school anatomy professor, and took a non-nursing class on death and dying with a hospital chaplain. The chaplain had us write poetry and short stories. I wrote a poem on the stultifying effects of nursing school, on the many ways the educational approach was dehumanizing, and how my nursing instructors seemed intent on extinguishing any compassion or empathy we came into school with. I delighted in words again and got excited when I realized the word "limbo" and the limbic system of the brain had a common root derivation: the region on the border of Hell. I had learned that the limbic system is the deepest and evolutionarily oldest part of the human brain, and is responsible for regulation of emotion, especially of fear. It was also responsible for memory, hunger, sexuality, and decision making. And limbo was what I felt myself suspended within, like the fruit in church supper Jell-O salads. Limbo was the dissonance of the South I had swallowed as a child. Limbo was the ambivalence I felt in my life about relationships, about my choice of careers, even about where I wanted to live. I desperately wanted out of the paralyzing limbo.

I went to a lecture on medical humanism by a Georgetown University professor and was mesmerized by his talk. Afterwards I was more convinced I could make nursing work for me as a career, a career combined with reflection, moral reasoning, and continued learning through reading and reflective writing. I wrote in my journal, "When I'm feeling ambitious and zealous, nursing seems old and stale and a hindrance to me as a person. When I'm feeling religious and humble, I can't imagine a higher calling than being a nurse. There's so much to do in this world, even right here in Richmond." I was drawn to working with homeless people in my hometown.

I became interested in homelessness while at Oberlin. In my sophomore year I took a psychology course on child abuse that included a practicum working with children at Green Acres Children's Home, which was located on the outskirts of Oberlin. My professor paired each of us with a young person who had survived some form of abuse or neglect. I was matched with Sherrie, a twelve-year-old girl who lived in the group home because she had recently run away from her foster home. Physically and sexually abused, she had already lived in five different foster homes and two group homes. I was Sherrie's big sister for the next two years, riding the bus to pick her up at the group home, taking her back to the small college town, buying her ice cream or lunch in a diner, teaching her to swim in the Oberlin pool, or just hanging out with her talking about normal girl stuff like boys and clothes. I never asked about her past because we were encouraged not to, but as I got to know Sherrie, she told me how sad she was that she couldn't live with her mother anymore. At the time it struck me as odd that, despite all the abuse, she still loved her mother.

When I was in graduate school at Harvard, I decided to heed the advice of my professor of health policy and get some work experience in community health. I worked part-time as a home health aide through an agency in Boston. My main patient was a twenty-nine-year-old black woman who was homeless, or rather had been homeless until she was hit by a car and ended up in the hospital. As she was recovering from a broken leg, she stayed at her aunt's small apartment in Roxbury. It was my first experience using food stamps. She would give me her food stamps and a grocery list and I'd go down to the small corner market with bars on its windows. As I traded the scrip for food, people in the store looked at me funny and seemed to wonder why a clean-cut white girl in khaki pants and a button-down shirt was using food stamps.

Now that I was living in Richmond, I saw an increasing number of homeless people on the streets. I had some patients in MCV hospital who were homeless, and I walked past clusters of homeless adults, including some homeless women, when I walked back and forth from my dorm to the nursing school building and the hospital on Broad Street.

I started volunteering at a small storefront free clinic for the homeless located in downtown Richmond on Broad Street, not far from MCV hospital. CrossOver Clinic had been started by a lung doctor, Cullen Rivers, and his Presbyterian church friend, the Reverend Judson "Buddy" Childress. The clinic had ties to the work of Jerry Falwell and the Moral Majority. Buddy had been a life insurance salesman before going to seminary. He was tall and had the physique of a former linebacker, now teetering on the edge of pudginess, with a doughy face punctuated by a boxer's broad nose. He didn't have a church. His ministry was to business and professional people, as he often said, "linking the talents and resources of suburban Richmond to the needs of the inner-city poor." Cullen and Buddy had started a free Saturday health clinic out of a storefront African-American Apostolic church, the Word of Life Assembly of God, in downtown Richmond.

Balding, with long, thin sideburns as bookends around a serious, intelligent-looking face and large eyes, Cullen was medium height, thin, and prone to wearing cardigans. He was practical and caring in a genuine way, one of those people with a quiet personal faith you wouldn't mind having yourself, even if you were agnostic. Some people have a loud, clanging sandwich board, standing on the street corner yelling at you through a megaphone, obnoxious sort of faith. But Cullen wasn't like that. It was one of the things that attracted me to CrossOver Clinic—that, and the fact that he and Buddy were trying to provide basic health care for free to poor people.

I had been married for two years to Charles, a sort-of-arranged marriage dictated by my parents, and especially by my mother. Charles was from a respectable Presbyterian family. When I met him he was finishing two years of study at a Pentecostal Bible college in Upstate New York, and he was starting seminary in Richmond. Ministers continued to run rampant in my family; by then I also had two brothers-in-law who were ministers or the sons of missionaries. Charles and I talked about doing future missionary work in other countries once he'd finished seminary. Through my work at CrossOver, I started realizing there was missions-type work to be done in my own hometown. I liked the feeling of things falling into place in my life, of the dissonance and ambivalence lessening, of finally figuring out who I was and what I wanted to do.

I went to Bible study meetings with my husband. I dressed in dowdy, demure clothes, sat in stiff-backed chairs, sipped tea from flowered china cups, and listened to the discussion and prayers without saying much. I felt numb and detached and mute, and knew I was playing the role of pious, young, Southern Christian wife.

On our first wedding anniversary, I carefully thawed the carrot cake with cream cheese frosting that my mother had saved from our wedding. I made dinner for Charles and afterwards I served the slices of cake on our lavender-blue flowered wedding china.

"Here's the cake. Happy anniversary, sweetie," I said as I stood beside his chair and presented him with the piece of cake. When he took the plate, I quickly pushed his face into the cake, laughing when he got a face full of icing.

"Jo, why did you do that?" he asked, grabbing his napkin to wipe his face, looking up at me with a scowl through the thick white icing.

"I have no idea. I just thought it would be funny somehow. The cake tastes like freezer burn anyway," I replied, turning back to the sink to do the dishes.

The years blended together. I finished nursing school and worked two part-time nursing jobs while going to graduate school to become a nurse practitioner. I continued to volunteer with CrossOver Clinic on weekends and did my master's thesis on the health of Richmond's homeless population. I knew it was a population I wanted to work with. Buddy and Cullen wanted to expand the work of Cross-Over, so I created my first job as a nurse practitioner, running the CrossOver Clinic at the newly opened Richmond Street Center.

Buddy and Cullen did much of the behind-the-scenes administrative work to keep the clinic running. It helped that Cullen was my main medical backup person and was available to me by phone for questions; he exuded an unflappable, competent demeanor, as well as respect for me as a nurse practitioner. I had two strikes against my credibility. Along with the fact that I looked younger than I was, nurse practitioners were a novelty. The role was less than twenty years old, and it was a role not always accepted by the conservative medical establishment. Buddy had good business sense and knew how to work his connections to get money and supplies for the clinic. He convinced a group of local nuns, the Sisters of Bon Secours, to pay my salary.

Over the first few months of working at CrossOver Clinic, I got to know the staff from the two main agencies at the Street Center, Freedom House and The Daily Planet. We all worked together to provide the necessarily-connected health and social services that homeless people needed.

Freedom House was modeled after Dorothy Day's Catholic Worker "houses of hospitality" and run by Larry Pagnoni, an energetic Catholic guy with the aura of a priest in jeans. He was twenty-four years old when the Street Center opened and he had spent a week or so living on the streets to find out what it was like. In talks he gave to church groups or to the local media, he liked to pull out a key that he always had on his key chain. He said the key was to his parents' house. He pointed out that most people who aren't homeless have a literal or figurative key to a family member's house; they have the necessary family connections as a fallback when times got tough, connections to ensure that they won't end up homeless.

The Freedom House staff members were all mostly young, college educated, and from middle-class families. They lived in voluntary poverty in run-down housing in Jackson Ward near the Street Center. In a way, they embraced poverty and homelessness. They got their clothing from the church clothing closets and their food from the food banks. None of them had medical insurance, so they relied on charity medical care, including what I provided at CrossOver Clinic. At the time, that didn't seem odd to me. Sometimes I couldn't tell who was a Freedom House staff person and who was a homeless client. I think Larry liked it that way. The Freedom House philosophy was similar to liberation theology, with God loving the poor and the homeless preferentially, and with Christians called to fight for social justice by whatever means necessary, short of actual physical fighting.

In contrast, The Daily Planet was a drug, alcohol, and mental health service agency, mainly composed of social workers, with its roots in the 1960s counterculture. They got their start by counseling young people coming down off bad trips from street drugs. There were many such young people hanging out around the nearby Monroe Park campus of VCU. The Daily Planet took its name from Clark Kent's newspaper of comic-book fame; drug-tripping clients said they felt like Superman when they came out of phone booths after talking with agency staff. Sheila Crowley, the head of The Daily Planet, repeated this story often, followed by a rumbling laugh. She was in her mid-thirties, tough, and staunchly feminist, with long wavy hair and oversized glasses and long-sleeved shirts rolled up over her muscular biceps. Sheila looked uncannily like photos I had seen of a young Gloria Steinem. As if she were a scrappy pit bull with a shredded ear I might see loose on the street downtown, I gave Sheila a wide berth at first. I could easily differentiate the Planet staff from the consumers; the staff members were all like Sheila. The women staff members were zealous white feminists and the men were Deadhead-type hippies. They were not big fans of any organized religion, but they were tolerant of the varieties of Christian do-gooders they now found themselves working with, for the common cause of combating homelessness.

When the Street Center opened in April 1986, homelessness was getting extensive national and local attention, with almost daily newspaper and TV news coverage. In May of that year, USA for Africa teamed up with Coca-Cola to sponsor Hands Across America to raise money for "fighting hunger and homelessness." They had thousands of people hold hands for fifteen minutes in cities across the nation. President Reagan joined in the hand-holding from the White House, reportedly shamed into doing it by his daughter. There was a sense that homelessness, at least this new version of homelessness, could be cured.

As a group, people who were homeless were called street people; they were poverty made visible on the streets and sidewalks. Homeless people, mostly in the form of older alcoholic men, had been part of the American urban scene for a long time. They had been called vagrants, paupers, hobos, and bums. What was new was a combination of the sheer number of homeless people and the changing face of homelessness. There were now women, younger people, and entire families living on the streets. Homelessness was portrayed as a national disgrace, and the urban housing market crisis and government inaction were mostly to blame. People talked about upstream measures and prevention of homelessness, but in a fuzzy, idealistic way, such as ending poverty and increasing low-income housing. There was frequent mention of deinstitutionalization, the effort to get mentally ill and mentally retarded adults out of long-term mental hospitals and back out into the community. This was a laudable idea stemming from civil rights era of the 1960s, but one that hadn't worked out so well. Many of the people who had been in institutions, such as dreadlocked Louie, needed permanent supervised housing and on-site help with counseling and medication. That combination was scarce to nonexistent, and the services that did exist were underfunded and understaffed. Rising numbers of Vietnam vets, who had untreated post-traumatic stress disorder and who had become hooked on heroin or alcohol while in the Army, were now homeless. Most were men in their early thirties, at the time of their lives when they should have been settling down and raising a family, but they had been left behind.

All of us service providers at the Street Center believed in our grand cause. Homeless advocates such as Sheila pointed out that homelessness wasn't as big a problem in Richmond as it was in large cities like New York, and if our community acted fast enough we could prevent it from getting out of control. We had a barely murmured, mostly unspoken code of talking up the numbers of the homeless we were serving, while simultaneously talking down any individual vulnerabilities of homeless people, vulnerabilities such as mental illness and substance abuse. We feared that would fuel a backlash of public sentiment against homeless people. We had a vested interest in sustaining the funding for our agencies, for the homeless people we were serving, and for our own jobs. We would say we were trying to work ourselves out of a job, but I don't think any of us actually believed that.

Although I wasn't sure anyone would come to the clinic when it first opened, within the first month I had seen fifty different patients for eighty-one clinic visits (meaning that some patients were returning to the clinic for follow-up visits). After the second month I had seen one hundred nineteen patients for two hundred and fifty visits, and so it grew, all out of our one-room clinic. By the end of our first year of operation, I had seen over sixteen hundred patients for close to four thousand visits. I didn't need to exaggerate the numbers of people I was seeing. I was treating everyone from newborn babies and their moms to homeless men in their seventies. The majority of patients were homeless single men in their late twenties who had injuries and skin infections from fights or from life on the streets. We had clearly outgrown our clinic space, and by the end of the first year, the clinic moved down the hall to a new addition to the Street Center overlooking the back parking lot. We now had two exam rooms, a dental clinic room, an office, and a waiting room, but I was still the only employee.

Many of the clinic patients were young African-American men from Richmond who had burned bridges with family and ended up on the streets. The crack cocaine epidemic was beginning to reach Richmond from Washington, DC and Baltimore, bringing with it a rising murder rate. Its violence would soon spill over into the Street Center. Some of my patients were not strictly homeless. They were adults with stable chronic mental illness or marginally functional developmental delay, then called mental retardation, who lived in supervised group homes nearby. They moved in and out of homelessness.

Working at the Street Center Clinic in my first nurse practitioner job was either ambitious or ill-conceived, and I often thought it was both on the same day. I learned as I went along. After a few months working at the Street Center I no longer freaked out when I saw scabies or crabs, gangrene or schizophrenia. I consulted with Cullen by phone at least once a day, although he didn't see much of these types of health issues in his private, affluent West End practice. He and Randy Hensen, a family physician, would alternate coming in on Saturdays to see the more medically complicated patients, like those who had uncontrolled hypertension or advanced kidney disease. With the new clinic addition, we had volunteer dentists on Saturdays to provide basic dental care.

The worst thing I did that first year was to give penicillin to a patient who forgot to mention, and whom I forgot to ask, whether he'd already had a severe allergic reaction to it sometime in the past. Luckily, he got back to the clinic in time for me to give him a shot of adrenaline and call the ambulance. As we waited for the medics to arrive, I monitored his status, while trying to appear calm, as the natural adrenaline surged through my own body. He was checked out at the hospital and released. I realized the level of responsibility I had, but also that I was not working completely alone: there was backup medical care available for real emergencies. It was the nonemergency medical care that was harder for homeless people to find.

The first year, I had a lot of freedom in the job, including latitude to improvise different approaches to providing health care for the population, such as conducting group tuberculosis screenings during the meals downstairs in the Street Center. This freedom was based on my relationship of trust with Cullen, the medical director. He kept reassuring me that he trusted my judgment to do what was right. But my freedom also depended on a rigid role I had to play, and which I played well, for Buddy and the board of directors. I carefully prepared typewritten monthly reports for the board, describing my clinic activities, the numbers of patients seen, and outreach and fundraising activities I had done. I included statements such as "God continues to use this clinic to reach many people with many and diverse needs," and signed off with "Respectfully submitted." This deferential approach was expected of me. I had grown up in the South; I knew how to be a proper Southern woman and at that point I was, or pretended to be, because it was easier that way.

As our patient volume grew, along with the medical complexities of the patients, I became more vocal in asking for help. In response, our clinic attracted an interesting assortment of volunteer physicians. Many of them only stayed a few weeks or months. They got frustrated with the homeless patients who wouldn't do what they told them to do. Some physicians asked if by volunteering they would be eligible for a tax deduction for charity. When the answer was no, they didn't come at all. Others stuck around longer, like an infectious-disease doctor from MCV hospital and a private-practice psychiatrist. The infectious-disease physician was helpful since the HIV/AIDS and tuberculosis epidemics were hitting our clinic population especially hard. He had helped with the medical care for Lee. While Lee was my first patient to die of AIDS, there would be many others after him.

The volunteer psychiatrist—I'll call him Dr. D—was pragmatic and liked the idea of street-based psychiatry and reality therapy, focusing on solutions in the here and now as opposed to plumbing the depths of childhood for the origins of life's troubles. It sounded like a good approach for our population. Dr. D was in his late twenties, just out of medical residency, a thin, quirky white guy wearing baggy Southern prep khakis and pastel oxford cloth shirts rolled up at the sleeves, bony elbows sticking out. He had fuzzy pale-red hair and a little-boy face drowned by round tortoise-shell framed eyeglasses. His eyeglasses mesmerized me, as they were constantly sliding down his blunt nose before he pushed them up quickly with an index finger. I watched the glasses, wondering if they ever fell off his face.

The first time I met Dr. D, he sauntered into my office as I was talking to a nursing student doing her community health rotation with me. It was early September of 1987, my second year at CrossOver Clinic.

"You know, I don't really like nurse practitioners. All the ones I've ever met have a problem with men and with doctors, so they end up having a problem with me." He leaned back against the sink, arms crossed, grinning, looking at me over the rims of his glasses as he pushed them back up onto the bridge of his nose. I wasn't sure whether he was flirting with me, or if it was part of some strange psychological test, or both.

I was beginning to wear makeup and was dressing less like a matronly missionary. Men were noticing me more often and it was both exciting and disconcerting. I was also a new mother; my son, Jonathan, had been born that May. Jonathan was a healthy, happy baby. My husband was still in seminary and now the three of us were crammed into the small second-floor apartment of a house in Ginter Park. Sometimes our small kitchen was strewn with clotheslines full of drying cloth diapers.

My marriage was showing the first hints of serious fraying, but I chalked it up to the stress of being new parents. I had seriously underestimated the amount of work it took to be a new mom while also holding down a full-time job. Charles helped out with the baby when he wasn't in classes. He was a caring and gentle father. Sometimes when I came home from work, Charles was making dinner while singing spiritual songs to Jonathan who was strapped to Charles's front in a baby carrier. We relied on my salary, which at $20,000 was just above the poverty line. I liked to think I was still happily married; I needed to be happily married since I was working for a conservative Christian agency. Although it was not explicitly stated in my job description—maybe because I had written my own job description—it was understood that I had been hired because I was perceived to be a proper Southern Christian wife and nurse.

With my back to Dr. D, I shuffled patient charts on my desk, handed one to the student nurse, and told her to read through it in the next room. I looked at more papers while trying to think of a way to respond to Dr. D's statement, and then decided to ignore it and orient him to the clinic instead. We got along fine and he never brought up his bias against nurse practitioners again. He came to the clinic twice a month for over six months to consult on our most complex patients with mental health issues. After being in the exam room trying to talk with a young white mother from the nearby family emergency shelter—she had her four hyperactive children, all under the age of six, with her that day—he walked into my office, breathless and clutching his eyeglasses in his hand. He asked me for a large net to throw over them. By that time I was more discerning of his humor and knew he was only half kidding: he'd probably use the net if I had one.

After a few visits with this family, Dr. D decided they needed more help than he could provide, so he turned his attention to Louie, who still occasionally wandered into clinic for Band-Aids for blisters on his feet. At least Louie told me they were for his feet, or rather Louie pointed to his feet when I asked him what the Band-Aids were for. He wouldn't let me look at the blisters and I didn't force the issue. I was trying to build up enough trust with Louie so he'd eventually let me help with his other health problems. Body lice were crawling around on the seams of his clothes. His schizophrenia was bad enough and his thoughts were so disorganized that he didn't seem to notice the lice. I never saw him scratching where the bugs must have been biting him incessantly. That can happen with his type of schizophrenia. People lose touch with reality to such an extent that they disconnect from many bodily sensations, like when they dress in down coats in the summer heat and don't recognize when they are sick. But I also didn't push the issue of the Band-Aids with Louie, because I knew he was unpredictable and could become violent.

I had experienced it myself. Six months before, at the end of a Saturday clinic when I was closing up and everyone had left, Louie walked in and carefully arranged his bedding and backpack in a corner of the clinic waiting room, over near the elevator. I was seven months pregnant at the time, exhausted, and wanted to go home and take a nap. I tried to convince Louie to leave, saying I had to lock up and he couldn't stay in the clinic. Even though I said this nicely, I forgot and positioned myself between Louie and the exit door. This is never a good idea with a person who has mental health issues and who is agitated, because he or she needs an easy escape route. Louie lunged at me, screaming and gesticulating wildly with both hands. I was shocked and terrified—shocked because I had never seen him act like this, and terrified because I feared for my baby's life as well as for my own. The clinic was empty except for Louie and me. Luckily, Sheila was working in her office nearby and heard Louie's yelling. She ran out and quickly calmed Louie, convincing him to leave the clinic space. She did this so easily, I felt both relieved and incompetent. After Louie left, Sheila hugged me and I began sobbing, glad that the clinic was empty, as I did not want any of the staff or patients to see me crying. I was wary of Louie after that. And of Sheila. I was embarrassed that she'd had to rescue me. I also had moments of wondering if I was putting myself—and my baby—in too much physical danger by working at the Street Center.

After Dr. D had taken a special interest in him, Louie's lice got so bad that the social workers and staff of the Street

Center considered banning him from services for fear he was spreading lice to other clients and staff. He even had pubic lice, otherwise known as crabs, covering his eyelashes. This was something I had only seen in textbooks. The lice looked like sooty snowflakes dusting his eyes. Clients were complaining about him and staff didn't want to go near him. Even though lice don't spread disease, Louie was becoming a public health threat. He refused to take a shower or have his lice treated, and we couldn't force him to do either. Sheila called for an informal Street Center staff meeting.

"It's getting bad enough with Louie that we need to do something, but I'm not sure what," Sheila said, starting off the meeting. There were six or so of us there, including social workers from The Daily Planet, several of the Freedom House staff who worked most closely with Louie, and myself.

"What are our options?" the Freedom House shower supervisor asked.

"We can ban him from services and hope that gets him to start taking care of himself so he can come back. We'd need to decide on the conditions for him returning and make sure he understands what those are, which may be hard to do. Or, if we really think he is a danger to himself, we can try to get him green warranted. That's not easy and I don't like doing it unless there's no other option."

To have someone involuntarily committed to a mental hospital for treatment was tricky. In Virginia, it was a process that necessitated a judge's order and was called a green warrant. No one at that point could tell me why it was called a green warrant. Later, when I had to get a green warrant on another patient and was sent a copy for his chart, I found out the form was typed on dull green paper, the color of hospital walls. To get a green warrant meant you had to prove the person was a credible threat to himself or herself or to someone else. Then the person could be taken against his or her will to a mental unit at a hospital for evaluation, observation, and treatment. Suicide and homicide threats were fairly clear-cut, but for someone like Louie it wasn't as easy.

"Well, he mainly has lice right now. He won't let me do a tuberculosis test. If he had active TB we could get him hospitalized for that, but lice isn't in the same category. Our psychiatrist has been seeing him a lot lately. I can call and ask his advice," I said.

Dr. D worked his professional contacts and got a court order to have Louie admitted to a local hospital. They figured out Louie's last name, and he stayed at the hospital for two weeks. When he returned to the Street Center I barely recognized him. Minus his dreadlocks and lice, he looked clean and acted sane. He didn't talk much more than usual, but what he said made sense and was quite intelligent. He even quoted poetry. We were all stunned at the transformation. At the hospital they had started Louie on Prolixin, a powerful antipsychotic medicine, and I was supposed to give him his monthly shots of it. The hospital had discharged him back to the street—to his dumpster shack behind the Street Center—as if it were a decent place to live. I am sure they would have said they did the best they could, and that's probably true given the circumstances and available resources.

For a few months Louie did well, stayed sane, and came in for his monthly Prolixin shot. I always made sure that I gave Louie his shot without putting myself between him and the door. Then he disappeared for several months, returning one day to the Street Center as disheveled and psychotic as before. Dr. D happened to be there a few days after Louie reappeared. He looked out of the window in my office and saw Louie behind the dumpster, busily setting up his makeshift home again.

"Jo, give me Louie's Prolixin and a syringe. I'm going out there and give him his shot." Still staring intently out of the window, he held out his hand behind his back, waving it in my direction.

"You're kidding, right?" I asked.

"No. I'm dead serious! Give me the medicine. I'll ask him first if he wants it, but I want the syringe ready in case he doesn't object."

I drew up the medicine in a syringe and handed it to him. "This is crazy, you know."

"Yeah, well, I'm a psychiatrist. I know crazy. He needs this medicine." He walked out the door with the syringe in his hand.

I gazed out of my office window at Louie in the empty parking lot: a square of lumpy pot-holed black asphalt, a large green dented metal dumpster on the far right corner, Louie's old doors and orange plastic sofas, all framed by the surrounding chain-link fence topped by curlicues of barbed wire and kudzu vines. The scene was laid out like a grungy movie set. I saw the psychiatrist enter stage right and approach Louie. Louie turned and faced Dr. D for what seemed like a minute or so. Then I saw Louie run off to the left with Dr. D in hot pursuit, waving the syringe over his head.

It was funny and sad wrapped up together, similar to dramas played out daily in the parking lot below my clinic window, where clients gathered to smoke and sneak gulps from bottles of booze sheathed in brown paper bags. Seeing it as a movie set was one way I got through the days. I parked my dingy tan Ford Escort station wagon in the back parking lot every morning, walked past the little knots of people, up the metal fire escape stairs attached to the outside of the building, and in the door to my third-floor clinic. From the top of the stairs I could see the guards patrolling the Virginia State Penitentiary grounds next door. Going through the main door of the Street Center off of Canal Street was overwhelming, with the open, dimly lit room full of tables and chairs, clouds of cigarette smoke, and the press of smelly bodies. The Daily Planet people called it the Living Room. If I went in that way I'd get stopped by various patients wanting me to look at their wounds, or to ask me about other health issues they were having, and I'd never get to the clinic. I also did not feel comfortable or safe downstairs.

Most days after the lunchtime clinic hours were over and I was working on charting, I'd close my office door, turn off the overhead fluorescent lights, sit in my swivel desk chair, put my feet up on a low filing cabinet, and gaze through the window at the sky and the treetops and tall gray towers of the nearby Jefferson Hotel. Clumps of kudzu waved in the breeze from the tops of the tulip poplar tree nearby. I tried to forget where I was for those moments, feeling closed off from the chaos of the Street Center that surrounded me. I had a small patch of sky and trees with no urban or human grime, or disease, or despair to mar it. I could breathe normally.

I wondered how long I'd be able to keep doing this work. It was physically and emotionally draining, and was at times dangerous. But I recognized that it was pushing me to become a better nurse practitioner, and was causing me to grow spiritually and emotionally. I thought about Larry's belief that God loves the poor preferentially and how it was more blessed to love the unlovable. I was finding it difficult to love some of my patients. I noticed myself passing judgment on their lifestyles and choices, like the ones who were drinking heavily, or doing drugs, or having too many children when they could barely take care of themselves.

Through my work at the Street Center I was learning more about my hometown and my home state—and more about myself.

Chapter Four

Relics

MY HOMETOWN OF RICHMOND, Virginia is a city anchored to its past by bronze and marble Confederate shrines of memory, by an undying devotion to the cult of the Lost Cause. I was born and raised in the furrowed, relic-strewn Civil War battlefields on the city's tattered eastern edge. A captive of its public schools, I was taught official Virginia history from textbooks approved by the First Families of Virginia. But I came to understand the shadowed history of my state by caring for its homeless outcasts.

These lessons began while I was in nursing school. The modern hospital of MCV curled around the former White House of the Confederacy like a lover. My clinical rotations were nearby in the crumbling brick former colored-only hospital, which then housed indigent and homeless patients as well as prisoners. Most of these patients were black, so I called it the almost-colored-only hospital. The prisoners, shackled to their beds and accompanied by brown-clad armed guards, were from the State Penitentiary located across town. One of my patients was a death-row inmate. When I spoon-fed him his medications, I was simultaneously afraid for my own safety and ashamed of being an accomplice to murder. I knew I was nursing him back to health only to return him so he could be killed by the state. I wanted to talk to him, ask about his family, about his life in and outside of prison, but the stone-faced armed guard loomed over me. I knew from experience not to discuss my ambivalent feelings with my nursing instructor. She considered these to be inappropriate topics. I wanted to finish nursing school as fast as I could, so I kept silent.

I wondered what the prisoners could see from their cells in the State Penitentiary. The area around the State Pen was an area I'd been taught to avoid—but not so much because of the prisoners. Oregon Hill, the neighborhood it was located in, was rumored to be as white, racist, inbred, and violent as an isolated Appalachian West Virginia hollow.

The residents of Oregon Hill were called hillbillies. Most were Scotch-Irish, descended from British bond servants who had moved to the area during Reconstruction to work at the Tredegar Iron Works and Albemarle Paper Company, both located along the James River. Darwin, in his introduction to *On the Origin of Species*, made reference to these settlers, called Crackers, who he said selectively bred black hogs because they were more resistant to disease than were white hogs—echoes of one of the many Southern justifications for slavery. At first Oregon Hill was a squatter's community, with people living on the land illegally. Then the settlers built cheap houses resembling coal-mining housing units.

Oregon Hill was a Richmond neighborhood that was easy to avoid: it was physically cut off from most of the city by the four-lane Downtown Expressway toll road. Urban planners, controlled by Richmond's white elite, catered to business interests in the downtown core. A 1930s city report targeted Oregon Hill for demolition, stating it contained the largest concentration of Richmond's cases of child and adult delinquency and disease. The nearby traditionally black neighborhood of Jackson Ward had also been slated for demolition for similar reasons. Both neighborhoods were seen as sources of moral contamination spreading like infection or mold through the city, sapping its vitality, keeping Richmond from becoming a leader in the New South. So the city built the Downtown Expressway in the 1970s, placing it through the worst slums, displacing thousands of impoverished blacks and whites and moving them to low-income housing projects. The Expressway wiped out half of Oregon Hill but didn't touch the State Penitentiary.

By the 1980s, the iron and paper mill industries along the river near Oregon Hill were closed, and the remaining neighborhood industry was the State Penitentiary. Built in 1800 on the crest of the hill overlooking the James River, the State Pen stood behind a tall cinder-block wall topped by shiny loops of barbed wire. It was an imposing fortress of gray concrete, almost windowless buildings.

———————————

One day in the late winter of 1986, I first visited the city-owned building being renovated for the Street Center. I'd been asked to look at the space designated for the small clinic I was to open and run. As I pulled into the building's deeply potholed parking lot, I was dismayed to realize it was located on the edge of Oregon Hill, just north of the State Penitentiary. Entering the three-story brick building for the first time, I felt as if I were crossing into the cave of the underworld. I questioned my sanity for wanting to work at a place like this.

Now that I was working at the Street Center, I was reminded of this every morning as I climbed the external fire escape staircase to my third-floor clinic. Pausing on the top landing, I looked over the recessed Downtown Expressway into the State Penitentiary compound and wondered if my former death-row patient was still alive. During my years working at the Street Center, four men were executed next door—at least one a year, usually during the hottest part of the summer. I had to drive through angry protests whenever there was an execution. White crowds seethed on the Oregon Hill side of the street shouting, "Fry the nigger!" while on the opposite side stood counter-protestors holding candles and softly singing "Amazing Grace." I didn't join them; I had a job to do. I knew that most of those executed were poor and black. They were killed at night, first strapped to a wooden chair with a hood over their face and then administered two 2,200-watt surges of electricity.

My patients joked about how the lights would dim throughout Oregon Hill when anyone was electrocuted. They also teased me about the chair I had in my office. It was a 1930s-era white enameled iron exam chair, donated by owners of a now-defunct tobacco processing plant with an employee's clinic. The arms of the chair swiveled sideways. Designed for ear, nose, and throat exams, the chair had a padded, adjustable metal clamp headrest. I used the odd-looking chair for taking vital signs and blood draws. Patients would often sit in it, place their heads back in the metal headrest, flap the iron chair arms back and forth, and call it Old Sparky. At first, their comments surprised me. Then it happened so often I shrugged it off, laughing along with them as if it were the first time I'd heard the joke—as if it were an appropriate joke. In the days leading up to an execution, the Street Center took on a carnival atmosphere. I chalked that up to remnants of racism and to the collective memory of lynching.

Virginia's deep-seated racism was embedded in state law and public health practice. Virginia's Racial Integrity Act of 1924 was an anti-miscegenation law spearheaded by Dr. Walter Plecker, a male physician and public health professional who was also a white supremacist. He was head of Virginia's Bureau of Vital Statistics, a division of the Virginia State Board of Health. The law mandated that a racial description of every person be recorded at birth, with babies sorted into one of two categories: white or colored (black or American Indian or anything else appearing non-white).

A companion to the Racial Integrity law, the Eugenical Sterilization Act, was also passed into Virginia law in 1924. This law was part of Social Darwinism, the Progressive Movement, and eugenics: bettering society through social and scientific engineering. Margaret Sanger, nurse and founder of Planned Parenthood, was a prominent leader in this movement. Virginia's Sterilization Act mandated involuntary sterilization of people institutionalized with mental retardation, severe mental illness, or epilepsy. The law also applied to prison inmates. They were all defectives or delinquents, viewed as a drain on society. People who were institutionalized and considered feebleminded included the shiftless poor, homeless people, juvenile delinquents, "chronic inebriates," and "oversexed women."

When Virginia established the Sterilization Act, eugen-icist doctors looked for a suitable test case to seal it into law. The doctor in charge of the Virginia State Colony for Epileptics and Feebleminded near Lynchburg, Virginia found his ideal candidates in three generations of Buck women. The widowed Mrs. Buck had been confined to the colony for having illegitimate children. One of her daughters, Carrie, had gotten pregnant at age sixteen, the result of a rape by a young man in her foster family, a fact that was covered up. A Red Cross nurse declared Carrie's daughter, Vivian, feebleminded at six months of age. The nurse reported that Vivian was "peculiar," with "a look about it that's not quite normal." Her assessments were used in official expert testimony. The head of the Virginia State Colony wanted to sterilize all three of the Buck women. The case went to the US Supreme Court, where the justices likened involuntary sterilization of degenerate offspring to state sanctioned immunization. Chief Justice Oliver Wendell Holmes, Jr. wrote, "Three generations of imbeciles are enough." The Supreme Court justices ruled in favor of Virginia, so the Buck women were sterilized—except for Vivian, who died while in foster care at age eight.

After the Supreme Court ruling, Virginia physicians aggressively pursued the Sterilization Act, giving Virginia the highest per capita rate of involuntary sterilization of the "feebleminded" and other undesirables. The Virginia Eugenical Sterilization Act wasn't completely repealed until 1979, just a few years before I became a nurse.

When I began work at the Richmond Street Center, I was only vaguely familiar with how my home state had tried not only to designate and separate the desirables from the undesirables, but also to extinguish the undesirables. A few of the Street Center activist social workers like

Sheila talked about it, but they were all Northerners, so I questioned their motives. It was disturbing, something I preferred not to think about. I was able to avoid thinking about these laws by relegating them to the category of relics from a past that didn't affect me—relics I didn't want to unearth. My work at the Street Center, especially with one patient named Sallie, changed that.

Sallie was twenty-five years old the afternoon she walked into clinic. It was at the beginning of my second year at the Street Center. Sallie was stocky, dressed in layers of boyish clothes with a greasy blue polyester baseball cap perched sideways on her head, covering her short red hair. She approached me silently, her head down, eyes on the floor as if she were looking for a lost coin. I caught myself looking down along with her. She began spewing a string of loud, tumbled words, but she stuttered so badly I didn't understand her.

"Ggggggot nkins? Got any nkins?" she asked, loudly, pacing back and forth in the doorway of the clinic.

"I'm sorry. I didn't catch that. What do you need?"

"You know—nkins, nikins," she repeated, pointing at her crotch.

"Oh! You need sanitary napkins. Hold on, I'll get you some. What's your name?" I asked as I rummaged in a supply closet.

"Sallie," she said, grabbing the box I gave her and walking hurriedly out the door.

This didn't qualify as an official patient encounter necessitating a patient chart, but I kept a log of 'almost' patient encounters and requests for supplies, so I needed Sallie's last name and age. I had seen Sallie hanging around the Street Center talking with one of the female social workers. Later that day the social worker told me Sallie had an IQ of forty-five and lived with her alcoholic, "mentally slow" mother in a run-down house in Oregon Hill a few blocks from the Street Center. Her mother controlled the monthly disability checks Sallie received.

Within the first year of opening, the Street Center had become a popular hangout for Richmond's marginally housed adults, including many who had mental retardation and mental illness. They moved around to live with different relatives, or they lived in cheap, moldering old downtown hotels. Others lived in Richmond's numerous group homes. Many of these homes were located less than a mile from the Street Center, a straight shot north up Belvidere Street where it turned into Chamberlayne Avenue. Chamberlayne had huge, stately old brick homes, now abandoned in the White Flight after school desegregation. The houses had been converted into group homes, women's shelters, a teen runaway shelter, and even an animal shelter. It was a social service ghetto.

Group homes had opened in response to deinstitution-alization efforts in the 1970s and early 1980s, as mentally retarded and chronically mentally ill people were moved out of state-run long-term-care institutions and back into the community. The idea, to provide supportive homelike living situations and community mental health care, was a good one. Most state long-term institutions were physically isolated, with rampant abuse and neglect of patients. But no one wanted group homes in their neighborhoods, so the homes ended up clustered in low-income or semi-industrial areas, places where the neighbors couldn't successfully fight the rezoning required. Most of the group homes in Richmond were poorly run, inadequately staffed, and lacked licensing oversight. There was also a deficit of community-based mental health and support services for the residents of group homes.

The Street Center social workers tried to be alert for clients like Sally with mental retardation or chronic mental illness, and to tie them in with alternative services. These clients were vulnerable to being preyed upon by the street-hardened homeless men in the center. The Street Center had free meals, lax rules, and staff members who were earnest, kind-hearted young people. The building was always bustling with activity, so it was a magnet for people like Sallie.

Sallie lived in the heart of Oregon Hill, located across Belvidere Street from the Street Center. By then I was no longer afraid to walk through Oregon Hill. Of course, it helped that I had the correct skin color to walk freely there. But I had discovered it was a nice place to retreat to on lunch breaks. In contrast with the Street Center's chaos, noise, and pungent smell of cigarette smoke combined with unwashed bodies, Oregon Hill's quiet, tree-shaded brick sidewalks were a welcome relief. There were rows of two-story wood houses with fading gray paint, sagging front porches, and Confederate flags draped across the windows as curtains. Some of the more run-down houses were rental units for VCU college students or the all-white 1980s punk bands. You could tell these houses by the piles of empty beer cans in the front yards, along with fraying upholstered couches and seats from old cars on the front porches. Mongrel dogs ran loose but were friendly. There was little traffic, except on Albemarle Street leading to the entrance of Hollywood Cemetery, which contained a ninety-foot stone pyramid monument surrounded by the graves of eighteen thousand Confederate soldiers.

For several months after her initial visit, Sallie came back to the clinic for more sanitary napkins, or for me to take care of small cuts, bruises, or splinters. She usually came in with a short, thin man with a large head, who she proudly introduced as Harold, her boyfriend. She repeated this every time she entered the clinic: "This's Harold. He's, he's, he's my BOYfriend!" followed by a beaming smile. I already knew Harold. He was a regular at our dental clinic. Harold was mentally slow—I didn't know his official IQ score—but he functioned at a higher level than Sallie did. He worked at a grocery store sweeping floors and he lived in one of the Chamberlayne Avenue group homes.

Harold had a misshaped face with a severely under-sized lower jaw and a perpetual grin revealing a set of teeth that resembled the bombed-out ruins of a city. The volunteer dentists who came to the Street Center Clinic on Saturdays told me they'd never seen a mouth as bad as Harold's. They took photographs to use in classes at the dental school. Harold's teeth were so badly decayed that the dentists had to replace them with full dentures. He was only twenty-eight at the time and was proud of his dentures. Harold insisted on giving me the stone mold of his lower jaw to use as a paperweight on my desk. He told me it was something to remember him by. Whenever he and Sallie came into clinic together, he would check to make sure I still had his teeth on my desk. Sallie would pick up the stone mold and pretend it was talking. For some reason her stuttering smoothed out and I could understand her better when she played ventriloquist. Harold grinned, showing off his dentures. But he always made sure Sallie returned his teeth to my desk.

Sallie got her health care at one of the MCV hospital clinics downtown, and she only came in for minor health complaints, so I didn't need to know her full medical history. I talked to Sallie in a light, breezy, stream-of-consciousness, almost playful way, as if she were a child. But, of course, she wasn't a child—she and I were about the same age. With Sallie, I learned to suspend basic assumptions about where she would go next in the conversation, and to follow her obtuse line of logic laced with random statements that were sometimes surprisingly insightful and other times hilarious. I came to understand her. She and Harold were sweet with each other. Although I knew to be careful of falling into the stereotype trap of viewing them as happy, childlike imbeciles, I did look forward to their visits. The couple was an antidote to the general bitterness of many of my homeless patients.

Idiot, cretin, feebleminded, moron, Mongoloid, retarded, funny-looking kid: all accepted medical terms at different times in history. More recently, the accepted terms are mental retardation, and intellectual or developmental disabilities. People in pediatrics sometimes use FLK for "funny-looking kid" to describe a baby or toddler whose face and head "just don't look right," but who don't have an identifiable genetic disorder. I remember the first time I encountered FLK on a child's medical chart in nursing school. I was shocked when my nursing instructor told me what it stood for. I was even more shocked that she didn't find the term offensive. FLK seems to be a throwback to phrenology—that pseudoscience of belief that low foreheads and bumps on the skull can foretell the criminal and devious propensities of individuals. FLK was what the Red Cross nurse had used to describe Carrie Buck's infant, Vivian, using it to label her feebleminded and in need of sterilization.

I had relatives with mental illness and mental retardation. My father's father and brother were tucked far away in the southern Appalachians of Tennessee: our family's living skeletons in the closet. I was told that my Uncle Charles was retarded, and that my grandmother was convinced it was because she'd fallen down a flight of stairs when she was pregnant. My maternal great-grandmother raised Uncle Charles on her cotton plantation in rural Georgia, so Charles had a thick Southern drawl and was the most openly racist of any of my relatives. He also had a serious speech impediment, talking as if he had a partially paralyzed mouth. He laughed loudly at his own jokes, startling me by suddenly reaching over and tickling me under the chin or slapping me on the arm. As a child, he frightened me; as a young adult, he embarrassed me. By then he lived with my grandmother and drove a delivery truck for a cousin's florist shop. With savantlike abilities in math, he had been tested at Emory hospital at age ten and assigned an IQ of seventy. He was considered feebleminded, trainable, and partially educable.

In my childhood, we went to my grandmother's house in Tennessee only at Easter, as if this were part of our family's annual pilgrimage of penance, death, and resurrection. Grandmother's house smelled of sick-sweet Easter lilies, boiled slimy collard greens, and Cimmerian dust from the dirt-floor basement's coal piles. My grandfather had a masklike face and lay in a tall four-posted bed staring at the ceiling. He talked infrequently, and when he did, it was in the staccato monosyllables of profound boredom. Poorly controlled diabetes and bipolar disorder had left him disabled. He frightened me more than Uncle Charles did. Grandfather was a lawyer but had lost his temper in court so many times that he was relegated to library legal research. After he lost that job in the Great Depression, he spent his days playing chess at the YMCA, while my loquacious grandmother sold *World Books* door-to-door. This was the oft-repeated family story. Grandfather died when I was six. Only my father went to his funeral.

Southerners are often stereotyped as inbred imbeciles. My Northern-born mother would tell me stories of my father's family when he wasn't around—about the mental retardation and mental illness that my father had been able to transcend by escaping to go to graduate school in New York City. Once there, my father was required to take speech therapy to get rid of his speech impediment: his Southern twang. Both of my parents continuously corrected my speech, determined to prevent me from developing a marked Southern accent. My mother examined the official IQ and academic test scores of all four of her children. Whenever she reviewed my report card, she'd declare I wasn't living up to my potential. With every "y'all" that slipped out and every "B" I obtained, I felt increasingly marked by the Southern blight. It wasn't until much later in life, while caring for my elderly mother as she was dying of cancer, that she informed me I was related to Varina Davis, First Lady of the Confederate States of America. My paternal great-great grandmother from the Georgia cotton plantation was Varina's first cousin, or something of the sort. I have not found an adequate place for that fact in my history.

The social worker brought Sallie into clinic one morning, pulled me aside, and said, "I'm worried about Sallie. She's throwing up in the downstairs bathroom every day. She can't be pregnant, can she?"

"Oh no. I hope not. I thought she couldn't get pregnant." I had assumed she had been sterilized. The truth is that I hoped she was sterilized.

I took Sallie into an exam room and asked her about the vomiting. She kept repeating it was the vitamins she took, that they were too big, so she choked and threw up. People in the feeding program downstairs insisted on serving up bowls of vitamins along with the meals.

"Sallie, would it be okay if you pee in a cup so I can check for infection or pregnancy?"

"Sure. What's pregcy?"

Oh God, please, she can't be pregnant, I thought.

Of course, she was. She couldn't remember when she'd last had her period, so I flipped through the pages of my patient logbook. I was dismayed to find that the last time she'd been in for sanitary pads was several months ago. When she got an ultrasound she was three months pregnant, too late for an abortion even if that had been an option.

Sallie's mother was her legal guardian and was anti-abortion. We also discovered she was anti–birth control of any kind. She claimed to not know that Sallie had a boyfriend and she accused the Street Center staff of allowing Sallie to get pregnant. Sallie's mother wanted to raise the baby, but she was a late-stage alcoholic. She threatened to go after Harold or his family for child support payments. All of this information I got through the social worker. We agreed: this was going to be a complicated case. We also agreed that this reinforced the negative stereotype of the mentally disabled—and of Oregon Hill residents—as reckless breeders destined to become a drain on public resources. Like with most stereotypes, there was a disquieting element of truth, along with oversimplification of a complex truth.

Sallie started going for regular prenatal visits at the MCV clinic downtown. My role was to make sure Sallie was taking her prenatal vitamins every day, which I hoped would help Sallie's baby avoid birth defects and a low IQ. I ground the pills and mixed the resulting powder with chocolate pudding to give to Sallie. As a nurse I was required by the state to report suspected child abuse and neglect, which this seemed headed toward. I didn't like being part of a system that could take children from their parents. I didn't like being an agent of social control, but I knew I had a duty to protect vulnerable children.

A simultaneous and distasteful part of my job was dealing with the childless, infertile white upper-middle-class Christian married women who hovered around our clinic in search of suitable babies to adopt. I was a mother by then, so I understood some of what it must feel like to desperately want a baby and not be able to have one. But the childless women—and there were several at any given time—were relentless. Wearing pastel cardigans and pearls, they would stop in to see me and drop off bizarre advertising materials: pages of contact information, glossy eight-by-ten formal studio photos of them beside their husbands, and written profiles declaring how well they could provide for a child. Their written profiles were as full of hyperbole as long Christmas letters. It felt obscene that they were shopping for babies at the Street Center and taking advantage of an already-marginalized population. Since our clinic was run by a conservative Evangelical Christian organization, I allowed the women to leave their advertisements. What the women didn't say directly but carefully implied was that they only wanted white babies. And they certainly didn't want to adopt a baby from a white mentally retarded couple, for fear the baby would also be mentally retarded.

Sallie's pregnancy was going well with no complications for either mother or baby. This surprised the social worker and me. Everything else about her pregnancy was complicated. The main unanswered question was who would care for Sallie's baby once it was born. Then there was the question of what should be done to prevent Sallie from having another pregnancy. Sallie didn't understand what pregnancy was, how it happened, or how to prevent it. None of the available temporary birth control options at the time were appropriate for Sally. She wasn't able to remember to take daily birth control pills and her mother wasn't reliable enough to remind her. The Depo shot and Norplant birth-control implants under the skin weren't yet available, and IUDs had been taken off the market because of the Dalkon Shield fiasco with its health complications and lawsuits. Doing a tubal ligation sterilization after Sallie gave birth seemed the best option. Sallie's mother agreed with this plan, but it also needed to go through layers of court approval. Laws in Virginia had changed by then to protect people from involuntary sterilization. The truth is I pushed hard for Sallie's sterilization. I told myself at the time I was doing it for Sallie's own good, but in reality I was thinking that three generations of imbeciles living in the Oregon Hill house were enough.

We all thought the father of Sallie's baby was Harold. Harold thought he was the father and was excited about the prospect of a baby. But Harold's family members were worried about possible child support payments, so they presented medical forms documenting Harold's sterilization procedure years ago. Sallie and Harold had been together for the past year and no one remembered seeing Sallie with any other man. Could Sallie have been raped? A possibility, but Sallie wasn't able to tell anyone.

Luckily Sallie's baby girl was healthy and looked white enough, so Sally's sister stepped in to raise the child. Sallie was sterilized after her delivery. She stayed in Oregon Hill with her alcoholic mother. Sally continued to walk into the Street Center Clinic beaming and announcing loudly that Harold was her boyfriend. Harold continued to shuffle in in behind her, quietly entering my office to check on the stone cast of his teeth still sitting on my desk.

I wish I could tell Harold that the stone mold of his teeth sits beside me on my desk as I write this. I wish I could tell myself why I have kept his teeth so long. Perhaps the stone mold of his teeth is a relic of unearthed truths I no longer want buried.

CHAPTER FIVE

Homeless Ghosts

A HALF MILE SOUTH of the Street Center was the wide James River, with its swift-moving rapids. Richmond was built on the falls of the river, which drops one hundred feet as it passes through the city. Along the riverbanks lived a group of my patients who called themselves the River Rats.

The River Rats consisted of a dozen or so adults, mostly men, with a few women who were married or otherwise attached to the men. All of them were white. They lived along the river on the edge of Oregon Hill. The River Rats ranged in age from twenty-six years old, to a man who said he was fifty-two but looked much older. Many of the River Rats lived together under a bridge by the river. A few ventured out onto a small island in the bend of the river in order to live in more seclusion. They were heavy drinkers who enjoyed the relative freedom of living outside on their own. The frat-party atmosphere permeated the area. On summer weekends the River Rats drank alongside the young, white, housed Richmonders who sunbathed on the flat rocks, or inner-tubed in the smaller rapids, floating coolers full of beer beside them. The River Rats drank outside year-round. They started in the morning, picking up momentum by evening. They were as loud and cackling as a flock of starlings. They got their money for booze from a variety of sources. Some of the older ones had monthly disability checks, others worked day-labor jobs, and several scoured the trash cans, alleys, and roadside ditches for discarded aluminum cans. They collected the cans and took them to the nearby R. J. Reynolds recycling center for money. Back then aluminum cans were going for a good price, and the recycling center was located close to the Street Center.

A few of the River Rats rode the rails. They hopped on and off the freight trains passing through Richmond. They were traditional hobos out of a different era. They had been to more parts of the country than most people had in their lifetimes—certainly more than I had been to. Several of them came to me with hand and knee abrasions from tumbling off a moving train and getting scraped up on the gravel bed of the railroad track. In my second year at the Street Center, one of my regular rail-riding patients was buried alive in an open coal car the morning after he'd celebrated his thirtieth birthday by getting more drunk than usual. His travel partner told me about it the next time he came into the clinic. He'd been sleeping in the woods instead of inside the coal car and hadn't awakened in time to get his friend out.

Richmond was at the crossroads of two major East Coast interstates, I-95 and I-64, as well as of two major freight train lines, so the city got a fair number of people traveling through, hitchhiking or riding the rails or the Greyhound bus, who stopped and got stuck, or stayed for whatever reason. They were like flotsam caught in swirling eddies of the river. There was discussion in the two local newspapers about whether the homeless people in Richmond were really from Richmond, or even from Virginia. Many of the newspaper articles featured interviews with homeless people who said they were from Baltimore or New York City or Philadelphia. The underlying implication was that many of the homeless people in Richmond were from the North; therefore, they were either invaders, or proof that the large Northern cities were dumping their problems on Richmond, taking advantage of Southern hospitality. Richmond was enabling felons, drug addicts, and lazy people who were homeless by choice. They would never be able to be recycled into productive citizens. Newspaper articles were more sympathetic to homeless people in Richmond who reported being from impoverished rural areas of Virginia or North Carolina. Whether they were black or white, they had been dealt a bad hand in life. They were our people and we took care of them.

Homelessness was an urban problem I associated with large, gritty urban areas like New York or Baltimore. I was surprised to see homelessness on such a large scale in my own hometown. The center of Richmond was decaying. Discarded carcasses of old buildings were everywhere. There were buildings with boarded-up windows and doors, charred remains of other buildings, people's belongings dumped in disheveled piles on the sidewalk curbside: evidence of evicted people, now homeless. Driving through the city at night you could catch glimpses of dark darting shadows or muffled flashes of a cigarette lighter, flashlight, or candle in some of the boarded-up houses. The shadows were squatters, homeless people—ghosts. Houses that were still legally lived-in showed signs of faded beauty. Stone cornices and intricate wooden lattices dangled loosely from front porches.

Along Belvidere Street near the Street Center, two blocks of Oregon Hill houses had been razed to make way for an expansion of the university. For over a year, to cordon off the construction site from sidewalk and street, the construction crew lined up old doors from the torn-down houses. They leaned the doors against temporary chain-link fences anchored by large concrete blocks; this made a long expanse of multicolored doors, which was as beautiful and shocking as a modern art installation. Sitting in my car at a stoplight on my way to and from work, I'd stare at the doors. I marveled at the deeply saturated red doors, wondering what sorts of rooms they had opened into. There were also a few doors that had obviously belonged to children's bedrooms. They were decorated with brightly colored Disney characters, like Donald Duck and Cinderella, and several had height and weight charts on them. I wondered if some of the doors had belonged to patients of mine who were now homeless. And I wondered what it must feel like to be a child and recognize the stickers from your old bedroom door as you were being dragged along the street by the hand toward the emergency shelter. I couldn't imagine my son's blue bedroom door lined up along the street.

In stark contrast to the dismantled and rotting parts of the inner city, there were patches of rebuilding and renovating. The biggest of these was the ill-fated $16 million glass-enclosed Sixth Street Marketplace spanning Broad Street. Built in 1986, the Marketplace was meant to bring back small businesses to the downtown core of Richmond.

It failed and was torn down less than twenty years later at a cost of $67 million. Closer to the Street Center was the grand Jefferson Hotel, built with tobacco money after the Civil War. It had been sitting empty for over a decade, although it was occasionally used as a movie location or to host high school proms. The grand staircase of polished marble was rumored to have been the model for the staircase in *Gone with the Wind*. My Lee-Davis High School senior prom had been held there as the hotel was closing. My prom date was my on-again, off-again high school boyfriend. He had a neatly trimmed blond beard and mustache and wore a baby-blue tux. I wore a periwinkle-blue polyester strapless dress my mother had sewn. We slow danced to the Eagles' *Hotel California*, and had our photos taken on the stairs. The red carpet was frayed and all of the rooms off the main lobby were boarded up. It was an eerie and sad place to have a prom. But it was an appropriate place to have my senior prom, since I knew I was soon escaping the worn-out South by moving to Ohio to go to college. The night of my prom I was hoping to leave the boyfriend and the South behind me forever.

By 1986 they had completed a $34 million renovation of the Jefferson, and the hotel was reopened simultaneously with the opening of the Street Center. The buildings were several blocks apart. Standing in front of the Street Center on Canal Street, the Jefferson loomed over the top of it: pale-gray marble against dark brick, majestic rich above outcast poor. At night the tall gray clock tower of the hotel glowed in the floodlights.

A major problem coming to Richmond from the North was crack cocaine. The first year that the Street Center was open, crack trickled in around us, since it was mainly available from New York, Baltimore, and Washington, DC.

Within a year it had permeated Richmond, concentrated in the poor black areas of Jackson Ward and Church Hill. With it came the now-familiar rise in the murder rate, and an increase in the number of babies born addicted, black men imprisoned, and neglected children sent to foster care. Violence increased at the Street Center. One person was bludgeoned with a baseball bat while he sat at dinner downstairs. Another man was stabbed in the back parking lot near Louie's dumpster. There were many other acts of violence at the Street Center, although none as severe. My mother started asking me if I really wanted to work there, if what I was doing was safe. Charles echoed her concerns. I assured them I was okay. The little multicolored top glass crack vials began dotting the river, washing up on the shore in amongst dead fish and tree branches.

Crack cocaine was not the drug of choice for the River Rats. They preferred alcohol. They drank Night Train, Boone's Farm, Wild Irish Rose wine, and Budweiser beer, and smoked pack after pack of Marlboro, Pall Mall, and Lucky Strike cigarettes. Many of them were three-pack-a-day smokers, the dream of Philip Morris advertisers. The 7-Eleven across from the Street Center was their main source for alcohol and cigarettes. Sometimes the River Rats and other clients from the Street Center would drink in the 7-Eleven parking lot and get in fights, and then the police would be called to break it up, arresting anyone who had an outstanding warrant.

Nancy and Terry were the core members of the River Rats. They said the name "River Rats" came from the VCU college students who sometimes taunted them, but they liked the derogatory term, so adopted it. They had lived under a bridge by the river for the past two years. When the river flooded or the weather got too cold, they would move to an abandoned house in Oregon Hill, but they preferred to be under the bridge. They were married and lived outside because they couldn't stay together in any of the shelters. The shelters were divided by gender, and the only family shelter was for mothers and children only: if there were fathers with them, they had to stay in a separate men's shelter. Nancy and Terry didn't like staying in shelters anyway because they couldn't keep their dog with them, and people stole their belongings. If they stayed at the shelter, they had to sleep with all their clothes and their shoes on at night, otherwise they might not have them in the morning. Nancy and Terry were both in their mid-fifties and were from peanut country south of Richmond, part of the Black Belt, the decaying core of Southern poverty.

Terry was a Vietnam vet with heart problems. He came to see me at the clinic for blood pressure checks and refills of his medications. Terry didn't like going to the nearby McGuire VA hospital, which was across the river on the south side of the city. He told me there were too many reminders of the war at McGuire, and vets worse off than he was. I noticed he was coming in for frequent refills of his nitroglycerin tablets for his angina, and thought I'd have to send him to a cardiologist for a reassessment. Maybe his heart problem was getting worse. It wasn't easy getting one of my patients an appointment to see a cardiologist and I didn't look forward to the series of pleading phone calls I'd have to make.

"Terry, what's going on with your nitro tabs? You're going through them too quickly, aren't you?" I asked the next time he and Nancy walked into clinic.

Nancy laughed, head down, shuffling her booted feet behind him.

"Yeah, you know, I just get these chest pains and have to take the pills," Terry replied, stone-faced, looking past me out the window.

"Aw, come on Terry. Tell her what you're really doing with them," Nancy said quietly.

"Oh shut up, will you?" Terry shot back at her, smiling as he said it.

I didn't think he could sell the tablets; they couldn't have much street value. Nitroglycerin wasn't like narcotics, but maybe it interacted with something else to give some sort of a high. I knew I was naive when it came to street drugs. I had done a clinical rotation at a West End Richmond inpatient drug and alcohol treatment center in my last year of graduate nursing school. While there, I learned about Alcoholics Anonymous, Narcotics Anonymous, alcoholic blackouts, and narcotics and alcohol abuse among doctors and nurses, but not about street drugs. It was a private-pay treatment center with a different clientele from the one I was working with at the Street Center. As a result, I often conferred with Ed Gurski, The Daily Planet's chemical-dependency counselor. Ed had an office on the same floor as the clinic, and was there when he wasn't doing street outreach. He often brought his clients in to see me.

Terry was quiet, looking down at his hands, inspecting his nails, which I noticed were full of dark red dirt.

"He throws 'em in the fire at night 'cause they explode like fireworks," Nancy said, laughing through a toothless, gaping mouth. Nancy had had all of her teeth removed, as she told me, "years ago because I didn't want to bother with them no more. Dang things kept getting infected and hurting, so I had the dentist yank 'em all out."

Dental care for our patients had been even harder to get than cardiology appointments. Most of our patients had poor nutrition, were heavy smokers, and had never had dental care. We now had volunteer dentists who came to our newly expanded clinic, which included a dental office.

The dentists had made Nancy a pair of dentures, as they had for Harold. She didn't like wearing them and carried them in her coat pocket until she needed to eat; then she'd pop the dentures into her mouth. She weighed less than ninety pounds with layers of clothes and heavy boots on. I gave her prenatal vitamins and encouraged her to take them with whatever meal of the day she managed to eat, hoping to counter some of the bad effects of all the alcohol she was consuming. She and Terry regularly sold plasma for money—at the same plasma center where Lee had possibly contracted HIV. Nancy wore a large beige trench coat year-round and filled the pockets with river rocks so she'd weigh enough to be able to sell her plasma. She looked like a shrunken, toothless, but happy ragdoll. Nancy had given me a hand-crocheted baby blanket when I was pregnant with my son. Knowing her lifestyle, along with the fact that I had treated her for lice several times, meant that while I was touched by the gesture, I also washed the blanket several times before putting it in my son's room.

"I can't give you pills just to throw in the fire, Terry. But I know you need them for your chest pain, so I'll give you enough for a month," I said, conjuring my most stern tone.

"Yeah you're right. It's just they make this really cool popping sound when you throw 'em in fire and people get a real kick out of it," Terry said, laughing, turning toward the main door of the clinic. Ed and an older man had just walked in.

"Hey there, Jake! How's it going?" Terry said, hitting the older man on the shoulder in greeting.

Jake was quiet, but smiled briefly in reply. Although dressed in patched and baggy clothes, he kept his handsome, rugged, chiseled-featured face up. With his full beard and proud demeanor, he resembled profiles of Robert E. Lee.

"Have a seat here a minute, Jake. I'm going to talk to the nurse and then I'll be back," Ed said, walking toward me while pointing to a seat in the waiting room for Jake.

"Jake here's a good friend of ours. He's a brother of mine from 'Nam. Take good care of him for us!" Terry shouted my way as he and Nancy waved and walked out of the clinic.

I had noticed Jake before although he'd never come to the clinic. When I drove into the Street Center parking lot in the mornings, I'd often seen him in the driver's seat of an old brown Impala parked there. The backseat of his car had neatly piled blankets, clothing, and paperback books, and he had a crow perched on the back of the front passenger seat. Sometimes the crow had a string tether tied to its leg and other times it hopped around freely inside the car. Many of my homeless patients had pets of various types— mostly dogs, sometimes cats. A few of the younger patients had rats or snakes or even crickets, but this was the first pet crow I had seen.

Ed ushered me into my office, closing the door. He was a slightly built, brusque, and fidgety man, but we got along well and were even getting to be friends.

"Jake has a leg wound he got in Vietnam, but it won't heal up. He's had an alcohol problem, but has been meeting with me and going to AA meetings regularly. He won't go to the VA for his leg, but he's agreed to let you take a look at it."

"All right. I'll see what I can do," I said. I picked up a new patient chart with the intake history forms and walked out to the waiting room.

"Hi, Jake, I'm Jo." I extended my hand.

"Pleased to meet you ma'am," he said with a heavy Southern drawl, standing up, and shaking my hand firmly, leaning forward with a slight bow of his head.

"Come on in the room here so we can talk about what's going on," I said, ushering him into one of the exam rooms.

I had recently moved into the new clinic space, built on the back of the Street Center. The clinic expansion had been delayed a few months because the builders discovered that the Street Center was built on unstable land from the old city dump. As they were digging to lay the new foundation, a giant sinkhole opened up, threatening to destabilize the entire Street Center building. The workers filled the sinkhole with concrete rubble from nearby building demolitions, and then they continued building the addition. The new clinic space was an improvement from the one room I started out in, but it had its limitations. The two exam rooms had no windows, no ventilation, and no sinks, since all of those had been beyond our budget.

Once in the room, in response to my questions, Jake told me he mostly lived in his car, which he parked on Tredegar Street under the Lee Bridge so he could be near his friends but also be alone. When he had enough gas he drove his car to the Street Center. He liked to be by himself, but said he stayed near the River Rats, who claimed him as one of their own. He had known Terry in the Army and liked him: "But the others down there I could do without." He said this in a reflective, slightly detached way, not with the superior, judgmental air with which some of my patients talked about fellow homeless people. Jake had a quiet, introspective manner, but he wasn't dark or brooding. During my first year of working at the Street Center I had developed a sort of internal Geiger counter for unsafe, unstable patients—patients like Louie. Jake didn't come across as dangerous. His clothes were old but clean and he kept his beard neatly trimmed. His beard was the only thing about his appearance that wasn't Army regulation.

"So, the counselor told me about a wound you have on your leg. Do you mind telling me about it?"

"Oh yeah. He wanted me to show it to you. It's gotten pretty bad. I thought I was taking care of it okay, but being outside I guess ain't so good for it. It smells real bad. I hate for you to have to look at it," he said, leaning over, touching the jeans covering the lower part of his leg.

"It'll be fine. Let me grab some supplies and bandages first though so I can fix it up while we're at it. I'll be right back."

I went to my office, which served as medication dispensary, lab, chart storage, and supply closet. Plus it had a sink. I filled a plastic foot basin with warm water, iodine, and hydrogen peroxide. This was the standard foot wash mixture I had learned from our volunteer podiatrist. I also grabbed vinyl gloves, a pair of new socks, and bandages of different sizes. I wasn't sure what to expect with Jake's leg wound.

I went back into the exam room with the foot basin and supplies, and spread out towels on the floor by his feet.

"We can soak both of your feet while we're at it. I brought you a pair of new socks if you want them. Sound okay?" I placed the basin on top of the towels and arranged the bandages on the exam table.

"Yeah, sure. That sounds good. My feet get pretty beat up. I don't always have gas for my car, so I end up walking." He started to untie his bootlaces.

I did a lot of foot care at the clinic, and we had volunteers who came in monthly to offer special foot clinics. Of course, it had its Biblical roots, but there was something about foot washing that most people found comforting and even pampering. I didn't believe in reflexology, but I knew that having your feet cared for could somehow make you feel better all over, even if it was just temporary. Almost all the homeless patients I saw had foot problems. They had to walk around town to get to different agencies, meal sites, and day-labor pools. They walked in the rain and the snow and the heat, usually in ill-fitting, secondhand shoes with dirty, holey socks, and carrying heavy backpacks. They got blisters and calluses, fungal infections, ingrown toenails, frostbite, and trench foot. After a year working at the Street Center, not much about foot care surprised me anymore.

Jake rolled up the bottom of his jeans and put his feet in the basin, wiggling his toes.

"Ah. That feels real good," he said, shooting me a brief, shy smile before looking back down at his feet.

I noticed he had a dirty bandage on the inside part of his lower right leg. As I looked more closely, I saw that it was made of folded white paper towel with pink chickens printed on it, loosely covered by a clear plastic bag and secured by scraps of silver duct tape. I began to smell something worse than the usual funky foot smell. He saw me inspecting the bandage.

"It's a sorry bandage. I had to use what I could scrounge up. It's been weeping a lot and getting my socks and pants all wet so I covered it up best I could."

"You did a good job. Resourceful. It's good to keep wounds covered up if they are oozing stuff." I tried to sound upbeat but not too cheerleader peppy. I was getting nervous about his leg.

As I pulled on a pair of gloves and started to undo the old bandage, Jake told me the leg wound began after he'd gotten a grenade burn in the final year of the Vietnam War. He'd been dealing with the wound for over a decade. The doctors told him he had bad circulation in the leg from the burn, so it might never completely heal.

"I'm just worried they're going to have to chop my leg off one of these days and I'll end up in a chair," he said, rubbing his bearded chin with one hand. "That's why I don't like going over to the VA. Seeing all those men in chairs bums me out."

The smell started to get worse once I had loosened the duct tape. It began to permeate the room and I had to turn my head away as I fought back the urge to vomit. I swallowed hard, inhaled deeply through my mouth, held my breath, and turned back toward Jake, smiling. I didn't want him to see me gagging. When I pulled away the plastic bag and the paper towel, I saw that his leg wound was at least as big as my palm, with ragged blackened edges, yellow fluid, and plump pearly white bumpy areas. I had seen similar wounds before—all except the white bumps—and as I leaned in to look at that area more closely, I saw them move.

Those are maggots! I thought. Luckily I didn't say it out loud and I didn't recoil. I had grown up in the country and had seen many maggots before, but only in dead, decomposing animals like squirrels or hunting dogs that had gotten killed on our camp property. I knew what they were, but at first I could not figure out how maggots had gotten in Jake's leg wound. Then it clicked. But how to ask this tactfully, without offending him, a question I had never asked a patient before:

"Jake, have you ever noticed that flies get into your leg wound?"

"Yeah, they're at it all the time, especially now with the weather being hot and all. Why? Do you see maggots in there? I can't feel 'em at all because that part of my leg is numb." He peered down at his leg, unfazed by my question.

I nodded and realized that I wasn't going to be able to handle it any longer with the door closed. I excused myself, saying I needed more supplies, and went to see if anyone was in the clinic waiting room. It was between clinic walk-in hours so no one was there. I closed the main clinic door, grabbed supplies, and went back to the exam room, leaving that door open for ventilation. I was able to pick out the maggots with tweezers, clean the wound with sterile salt water, and apply a clean dressing covered by an elastic bandage. Jake pulled on his new socks, tied his boots, then stood up, stomping his feet gently to settle his jeans in place.

"That feels a whole lot better. Thank you, ma'am." He reached for my hand to shake, again dipping his head in an elegant bow.

Jake came back daily for wound care. I expected the maggots to return. I knew that maggots had been part of medical treatment of soldier's wounds during the Civil War, and were being reconsidered as current, accepted treatment. Maggots from the common green bottle fly secrete a natural antibiotic and also eat dead and infected tissue in wounds, helping them heal. But I didn't want maggots in Jake's leg. The presence of maggots in Jake's wound reinforced the specter of death and decay permeating my life in Richmond.

Since I was seeing Jake regularly for wound care, over the next several months I got to know him better. He wasn't talkative, but began offering more information, at least about his current life. There was something about the daily ritual of foot care and wound cleaning that nudged him to talk. I learned to modulate my questions with his moods, knowing when to gently probe, when to back off, and when to be silent as he brooded. It was like falling into step beside him.

Jake told me about his pet crow named Blackie, how smart she was and what a good companion she was because she listened and didn't talk back. "She had a hurt wing when I found her but she let me splint it. Healed up crooked but she's real strong." Insomnia and nightmares plagued him, so he stayed up most nights reading paperback novels by flashlight. Mysteries were his favorite, as long as they didn't involve much killing. He didn't like sleeping outside because it reminded him of the war, so he stayed in his car, or in a vacant garage he'd found near the Hollywood Cemetery on the edge of the river. He liked the quiet of the cemetery and was able to sleep better there. The ceiling of the garage had old glow-in-the-dark stars and he could see his way around at night by their light. Jake had been homeless off and on ever since he was discharged from the US Army ten years ago: "I tried going home but it didn't work out." I didn't press for details. His face closed down as he said it. Jake had a classic case of the recently named post-traumatic stress disorder—PTSD. It had older names, including battle fatigue and shell shock. During the Civil War it had been called nostalgia or homesickness.

I knew about PTSD, but only in an abstract, clinical sense. At the time, I didn't realize I would develop it myself. I wish I had known then what I know now about PTSD, how it festers and flares inside while leaving no visible scars. Maybe I could have done more to help Jake. Maybe I could have seen that his PTSD was more destructive than his leg wound.

What I would never know firsthand was what it was like to be a chronically homeless war veteran. The media liked to focus on this segment of the homeless population: the long-term disabled homeless and the large number of Vietnam vets who were on the streets. After the Vietnam War was finally over, people in the United States wanted to forget about it, but the presence of homeless vets on the streets wouldn't allow them to. Even though there were many people—vets and civilians—who were homeless for a short time and quickly became housed again, they didn't make for a good newspaper article or TV news spot.

In 1987, Mitch Snyder at the Washington, DC Community for Creative Non Violence was getting a lot of media coverage for homelessness, and especially for homeless vets. The people at the Community for Creative Non Violence had started out protesting the Vietnam War, then turned to advocating for the Vietnam vets who were ending up homeless. Mitch had joined them, becoming their charismatic spokesman. He had slept outside the Library of Congress in the winter, along with Hollywood stars, for the "Grate American Sleep Out," and he had been fasting again for some sort of homeless cause during the summer I was taking care of Jake. Mitch was controversial, but he helped draw attention to the issue, and in July, President Reagan signed the Stewart B. McKinney Homeless Assistance Act. The McKinney Act sought to provide money to meet basic needs of the homeless. It placed a special emphasis on vulnerable populations, including disabled veterans like Jake. Three years after Reagan signed the McKinney Act, Mitch would hang himself in his room at the Community for Creative Non Violence shelter, close to the US Capitol Building. Some people said he was depressed over a soured relationship; others said he burned himself up with passion for the homeless.

After a month of treating Jake's leg wound, it was getting smaller, it didn't smell as badly, and the maggots didn't return. I was able to clean and dress his wound in the exam room with the door closed. I got him to come in between clinic walk-in hours because I was seeing an increasing number of patients. For my monthly clinic report to the

CrossOver board of directors in August that summer of 1987—my second summer at the clinic—I wrote: "I have had a difficult time keeping up with the demand for services. This past month is the first time in my fifteen months of working at the clinic when I have been very much overwhelmed physically, emotionally, and spiritually." I added that I either needed additional help in the clinic or I'd have to restrict the number of patients I was seeing. My son was an infant and I was nursing him at night, so I was chronically sleep-deprived. I knew some of my frustration and fatigue was from that. But the clinic statistics pointed to a bigger problem. In July of the second year of the clinic, I saw close to 250 patients for 470 patient visits. My patient load had doubled from the year before and I was still the only clinic employee. I continued signing my reports "Respectfully submitted," although I was not feeling as respectful as I had a year before.

At the Street Center Clinic I was seeing a mixture of people who were homeless, as well as people like Harold from the adult homes nearby, and the working poor from all over the city. The Street Center mandate was to provide services to people who were living on the street or in shelters: people who were literally homeless. Yet no other free primary care clinics or reduced-fee community health clinics existed in Richmond at the time. The only real medical safety net service besides our clinic was MCV. Many patients viewed it as large and impersonal, with long waits to get care. Word had gotten around that we would see anyone who needed our services, and that we provided free medications. The CrossOver board of directors discussed the idea of starting to charge patients a nominal fee for medications as a way of, as they said, "instilling more accountability." This fit with the growing public sentiment in Richmond that homeless service providers were "soft on street people" and were making it easy for more people to become and stay homeless. A conservative Christian Richmond woman who volunteered at a church-based homeless shelter was quoted by Mark Holmberg in a December 28, 1989 *Richmond Times-Dispatch* article, "Homeless By Choice," stating, "We're building a homeless boom. Homelessness has become a fad. I'm waiting for the T-shirt."

I pointed out to the CrossOver board members that the Street Center was such a forbidding, undesirable place for anyone who wasn't desperate and homeless that it served as an effective needs-based screening of patients. For the truly homeless, charging for medications would mean they would go without them and get sicker. There had been a few newspaper articles focusing on our clinic and its services. I had hoped the news coverage would help us find more volunteers, but instead, we just got more patients. Especially since I was seeing more patients than I could handle effectively, I wanted to restrict the clinic to the homeless.

The Daily Planet and Freedom House administrators were applying for a federal grant to get funding set aside by the McKinney Act for expanding and integrating services for the homeless population. This included the first big round of Health Care for the Homeless funding, which was specifically earmarked for clinics like ours. Buddy Childress and some others on the CrossOver board of directors wanted to redirect our clinic services to focus on the working poor, but they also wanted the grant funding in order to hire a full-time physician for the clinic. They didn't have anyone who wanted the physician job, but they were advertising it nationally. Tensions were building like thunderheads— mainly between Buddy and me—about the direction of the clinic. I still got along fine with the two backup physicians I worked with, and wished one of them would take the clinic physician job. But they both had lucrative private medical practices they weren't willing to give up. I wanted a change, but wasn't sure what it was. I needed help at the clinic but I also wanted to remain the clinic director. I knew that a physician would take over this role.

I was feeling restless at work and at home, wanting something more and chafing at the roles I found myself playing. Sometimes I felt that I was literally and figuratively putting Band-Aids on the problem of homelessness, patching people up, and sending them back out into a life that was breaking them again. I was frustrated that I couldn't do more to address the bigger issues that were causing homelessness. I also prayed that God would take away my restlessness: I viewed it as a sin at times. I was getting tired of that sort of black-and-white religious thinking—the type of thinking my husband had—but I wasn't ready to give it up myself. Through my work at the Street Center, I was getting to know people whose worldviews were wider than what I had allowed my own to become. They were similar to people I had known while in college at Oberlin, especially my Spanish House roommate who was a Marxist socialist Zionist feminist who protested something different almost every day. Our dorm room was full of protest signs. She gave up on trying to get me to join the protests.

I didn't want to be a Mitch Snyder—dying for homelessness—but I did want to do something more to help change the world for the better. And I didn't see much value in voluntarily becoming poor and homeless, like the Freedom House staff. I didn't have much time to contemplate these conflicts; I was just aware of them, like distant thunder.

One day in late August Jake didn't return to the clinic. I waited a few days, asked staff members at the Street Center if they'd seen him, and then went looking for him accompanied by street outreach workers from The Daily Planet. We knew Jake usually hung out with the River Rats during the day. That's how I found myself sitting under the Lee Bridge by the James River on an August afternoon.

"Ain't seen Jake in a while now. I think he might'a moved on down south," Terry mumbled, wafting a miasma of stale booze and cigarettes in my direction.

If Jake's best friend Terry didn't know where he was, I was stymied. Another "Lost to Follow-Up" in my patient file system. I hated not knowing how their stories ended.

The social worker from the outreach team was busy talking with Nancy about benefits paperwork. I tuned it out since it didn't involve me. It was hot under the bridge. The breeze had died down, thunder growing more distant as a storm passed south of us. The air under the bridge was still, humid, and dense. The fumes from the traffic overhead choked off any fresh air. As I struggled to breathe, I looked at my feet, at the rich red dust covering my bare toes and coating my sandals. Dark-green kudzu vines sprawled over the hillsides, climbed power lines and enveloped dead trees, making them look from a distance like old castle ruins. Down the hill from us lay the gray gravel-bed railroad tracks. The CSX train lines of mud-brown cars filled with black coal lumbered through, parallel to the Kanawah Canal and past the dark building of the Tredegar Iron Works. Beyond the railroad was a line of sycamore trees marking the edge of the broad river dotted with large flat rocks.

I gazed out over the churning river in front of me:

the Second Break Rapids and the fiercer Hollywood rapids surrounding Belle Isle, a mile-long sliver of an island. There were tents and blue tarps showing through the tree canopy of Belle Isle—other camps of the River Rats. Belle Isle had been the site of a Powhatan Indian fishing village, then a Union prisoner camp during the Civil War. There were still standing walls of the brick prison buildings on the island. During the Civil War, most of the prisoners stayed outside in small canvas tents. Many died of exposure or dysentery and had been buried in communal graves on the island.

I looked west to Hollywood Cemetery, perched serenely on a bluff nearby. The rolling contours of the cemetery were anchored by spiny-leaved holly trees, stately magnolias, and rusting black iron filigreed fences surrounding crumbling grave markers. I'd already looked for Jake near there, in the star-filled abandoned garage where he sometimes stayed. There'd been no sign of him.

As I contemplated the dust covering my feet, it occurred to me that Richmond is built on the bones of African slaves and Civil War soldiers, mixed with the communal bones of the Powhatan tribe. The land is heavy with the remains of the displaced.

It became heavier for me a few weeks later. Terry came into clinic one afternoon and said, "Got some bad news about Jake. Fishermen found him yesterday. His body washed up a ways on down river. Police say he didn't have no bullet holes or nothin'. Looks like he just up and drowned. You figure it was an accident?" Terry cocked his head to the side, wrinkled his brow, and peered at me through narrowed eyes. He still smelled of booze and cigarettes, mixed with layers of campfire smoke and sweat.

I nodded. "Yeah, probably so." I knew Jake never went swimming in the river, especially with his leg wound still open. A fair number of people drowned in the James River in Richmond every year, especially when they got drunk and slipped off the rocks into the rapids. More than likely Jake's memories had killed him. But I kept those thoughts to myself.

I said more softly, "I hope so." Not for any religious reasons. Jake wasn't Catholic, as far as I knew, and my own religious views didn't include damnation for suicides. It just seemed like such a waste. And I was replaying all of my interactions with Jake over the past few months, trying to remember any clues I'd missed about his state of mind.

"He was a really great guy," I said, then remembered: "Any idea what happened to Blackie?"

"Yeah. He let her go a month or so ago down there by the river near to Hollywood. Jake said it was time to let her go. Damn bird just eyed him once and flew on up the river like she'd never knowed him. Ungrateful crow!" He chuckled.

CHAPTER SIX

Confederate Chess

IN SEPTEMBER 1987, a month or so after Jake died, I was working late in the clinic. Bruce walked into my office holding a small curly-haired white dog in his arms.

"Nurse Jo, you got to help Scruffy! She got caught on some barbed wire down by the river and got tore up."

Bruce was cradling Scruffy in both arms like a baby, and Scruffy's belly was bloody. I looked at Bruce's pleading face and at the docile dog. Scruffy wagged her tail as I walked toward them.

"Bruce, I can't. I'm not a veterinarian."

"I can't afford no vet. It's just a scratch, so you can patch her up real easy."

I had a soft spot for Bruce. He was one of the River Rats. White-haired, shrunken, fond of wearing blue overalls, he reminded me of an Appalachian apple doll. I'd often see him on the sidewalks near the Street Center, pushing a rattling metal shopping cart full of aluminum cans, and a large puffed-out black plastic garbage bag, with Scruffy perched on top of the pile, wagging her tail. Bruce was so short that he couldn't see over the piles in his cart; he darted his head out from side to side to see where he was going. He leaned his body into pushing the cart, his arms fully extended. Bruce was a boisterous alcoholic, so usually the cart didn't go in a straight line. He liked to give away presents he kept buried inside the garbage bag: packs of Marlboro cigarettes smuggled out of the Philip Morris plant by a friend of his who worked there, and packages of Twinkies and bright-pink Sno Balls from the nearby Hostess factory. With his scraggly gray beard and the bag of presents, he was like a back-alley Santa. Bruce's dream was to get a trailer of his own where he could be left alone to drink until he died. He tried to save some of the money he was making from recycling aluminum cans, but he spent most of it on wine and presents, like the day-old Hostess products.

Bruce was one of the nicest of our regular patients at the clinic. Even when he got drunk, he wasn't mean: if anything, he got kinder and gentler. He didn't have a chip on his shoulder, didn't project an "I'm angry at the world for being given such a bum rap in life" attitude. Some of the clinic regulars were so weighed down by anger they staggered beneath it. Bruce shuffled. He was plain sweet. And I knew Scruffy was his main companion.

"Okay, I'll take a look," I said, glancing at my watch. Besides wanting to get home for dinner, I was thinking I could get in trouble for providing medical care to a dog. But I decided cleaning Scruffy's wound couldn't be against the law.

Bruce and I washed Scruffy's belly in the bathroom

sink. The scratch was shallow and didn't need stitches. I put antibiotic ointment on the wound, covered it with gauze, and wrapped a pink elastic bandage around her middle. I didn't want to use tape since she was so furry. With the bandage on, she looked even cuter than before. Scruffy had a similar demeanor to Bruce. She didn't squirm or growl when I cleaned her wound, and she licked my hand when I wrapped the bandage around her. I wondered if this docility, this lack of anger, was inborn or learned behavior, and if it was healthier to not rage against one's fate.

The following week I was busy with children needing back-to-school physicals. In the weeks leading up to and right after school started, I had many children brought in by their mothers. The school nurses sent them to me to get caught up on their immunizations. The children were young enough to be excited about going back to school, despite their fears of getting shots.

I could always tell fall was approaching by the children. They got increasingly restless as the summer went by. I did weekly outreach to the family emergency shelter a few blocks from the Street Center, stopping in to see if any of the women or their children had any health concerns. In late summer, whenever I entered the dark living room of the shelter from the hot bright sun, stepping into the tepid air of the struggling window air conditioners, I was temporarily blinded by the darkness. Children swirled around, small hands and arms circled my legs with laughter. The large forms of the mothers sat listlessly on the sagging couches. One of the mothers would bellow at the children, "Settle down now y'all! I can't hear myself think with you ole crazy-ass selves!" The shelter staff cowered in their office off to one side. In the shelter I only had space and supplies to be able to see the children for colds or rashes or minor injuries. They had to come to the Street Center Clinic in order to get their school physicals done and to get their shots. Their combination of energy and enthusiasm was a welcome change from the general down-and-out depressed demeanor of many of my adult patients. Also welcome was the happy rhythm of seasons marked by the rituals of school. For the older single adults, the seasons seemed to blur together in one uninterrupted miserable trudge around town in search of food and shelter.

That fall I was also busy supervising a group of nursing students doing their community health rotation at the clinic. I enjoyed teaching. Although I didn't get paid for it, I got to teach the way I wished community health had been taught to me. I went into nursing for community health, and was disappointed by how rigid my community health instructors had been. They insisted we wear heavy navy-blue cotton uniforms that reminded me of the humiliating one-piece gym suits I endured in high school. They also issued us decaying black leather nursing bags, stiff with age, metal closures sticky with green corrosion.

The instructors demonstrated what they called proper bag technique: how to open and extract contents. The bags crackled when opened, emitting a moldering smell, and refused to stay open, threatening to pinch your fingers when you reached inside. The contents included a portable blood pressure machine, glass thermometers, and a strange-looking black sling with a small spring-loaded weighing device attached to strings: a primitive baby scale. But it looked more like a kinky S&M torture device. I hid my nursing bag at home and never used it; my instructor threatened to fail me for insubordination. Now that I was teaching a community health clinical section, I had students wear normal street clothes and didn't issue nursing bags.

As a new mother, I could relate better to the mothers I was seeing in the shelter and in the clinic. I knew the anxiety over whether or not your child was progressing normally in growth and development, with the underlying question as to whether or not you were being a good enough mother. My son, Jonathan, was five months old that September and was a thriving, happy baby.

In clinic, the nursing students screened the preschool children for physical and mental development using simple techniques from the Denver Screening tool, like having the younger children take raisins out of small boxes, having older ones hop on one foot, and noting their drawing and vocabulary skills. The children's laughter filled the clinic as the mothers sat back and smiled. At that moment at least they knew they were good mothers.

Besides covering clinic and doing outreach to shelters, I also did fundraising activities, giving presentations to churches and community groups. I had been asked to give a presentation to the Richmond Academy of Medicine. It was their first meeting in the fall after summer break, and my talk was scheduled for after cocktails and a sit-down dinner. I was invited for the talk, but not for the cocktails or dinner. Knowing it was a conservative group, I wore my grandmother's pearl necklace, hand-sewn Laura Ashley flowered blouse, and navy-blue pinafore jumper. The blouse had a stand-up ruffle at the neck. I had my hair pushed back with a brown headband, and I wore thick-soled black Mary Janes with Velcro straps. I had notes for my talk on fifteen or so index cards, all carefully numbered in case I dropped them. I looked and felt like a church librarian. I wanted to appear serious, capable, and pious.

The dinner meeting was held in a private dining room in a building around the corner from the Skull and Bones

Restaurant, near MCV hospital. It was a stately colonial brick building, with a dark-green canvas awning over the entrance. Closely clipped bay trees in black iron urns flanked the front door. As I stood outside looking at the building to make sure I had the correct address, I felt a sense of foreboding, and had an urge to walk away. It wasn't nervousness so much as a repellent force field. The smell of wet dead leaves and acorns was strong. I turned the brass doorknob.

In the foyer was a cluster of men dressed in dark suits and bold, aggressive ties. They were holding glasses filled with amber fluid, talking and laughing boisterously. As I walked in, one of the older men turned, greeted me, and ushered me into a side room. Clearly I didn't belong. I was the only female inside a boys' club: a rich, exclusive boys' club. A rich, exclusive, *white* boys' club. The only non-white people I saw were black male waiters hurrying around and refilling the men's drinks.

Earlier that day I'd had to raid a jar of loose change to be able to buy gas to drive to work. One of my shoes had a hole in the sole. I reminded myself not to cross my legs when I sat down because I didn't want anyone to notice the hole. The man leading me into the room had burnished brown tasseled loafers on his feet. They looked new and expensive. The snatches of conversation I heard were about recent vacations with their families to Cape Hatteras or to Europe. They were giving me a $100 honorarium for my talk. The CrossOver doctors told me it was my money to use as I wished. I bought pocket-sized New Testaments to give to patients. It made me feel pious.

The room I was led into was dimly lit and cold, like a museum. People talked in hushed voices. It was a large boardroom with a heavy-legged wood table dominating the room, a Persian rug underneath, and a large crystal chandelier above. The table seated about thirty people, and there were men scattered around the perimeter of the room sitting in upholstered chairs. The drapes covering the tall windows were burgundy velvet. As I sat at the table, the floor-level brass heat registers blew in dusty air, sending little eddies of warmth under the table. On the wall opposite me, a built-in bookcase held leather-bound medical journals and a brass bust of Hippocrates. The room looked sterile, like a stage set.

I felt like a visitor watching a solemn religious ceremony in a foreign country. In the foyer, the men were loud and garrulous, but as they crossed the threshold into the boardroom, they lowered their voices. They seated themselves automatically by a secret code. I was introduced to the club's president, an older man sitting at the head of the table. An obsequious thin young white man hovered around him, nervously passing out meeting agendas. The sound of ambulance sirens punctuated the muffled sounds inside. Again, as if by some signal, the room quieted. There was silence. The leader cleared his throat, started the meeting, and introduced me in a resonant baritone voice.

I was careful what I said about the clinic, and especially how I described my role there as a nurse practitioner. One of the men asked about the types of health issues I was seeing, where I referred people for specialty care, and what sorts of donations would be most useful. The man who had ushered me into the room praised my work; I felt simultaneously embarrassed, flattered—and suspicious. Several of the older men seemed particularly interested in my role as a nurse practitioner. Did I diagnose health problems? Did I prescribe medications, and if so, which ones? And how exactly did I prescribe them? They asked these questions in the manner of a court cross-examination in front of a jury, darting brief, knowing glances at each other, smiling sardonically. I recognized the turf issues. The unasked question was, "Are you trying to be a doctor?" I pretended I didn't know what was behind their questions and was politely vague in my answers. It was a setting ripe for a Southern version of the drawing room dissembling of Edith Wharton, and in my demure Laura Ashley attire I thought I pulled it off.

At the time, our clinic was operating on $30,000 a year, which came to $5 per patient visit, and averaged $25 per patient per year. The clinic costs included my salary, malpractice insurance, medications, supplies, and our share of the utilities. Before the clinic opened, the main source of health care for Richmond's homeless people had been the MCV emergency room. The average cost of a visit to the emergency room was $120, and the cost to the health care system was at least twice that amount, since the hospital had to underwrite charity care. The fifty-five hundred patient visits per year I was seeing at the clinic translated to a total cost savings of $1.3 million per year. Of course, not all of my patient visits would necessarily be averted emergency room visits, but the majority would. I told the doctors our total clinic operating expenses and the number of patient visits. They were smart enough to do the math, and some leaned in together to quickly comment and shake their heads.

Nowhere in Virginia at the time was there a similar nurse-run clinic. There were several clinics for the homeless in Washington, DC, but they were staffed and led by doctors. I wondered why there were no nurse-run clinics in Virginia, but no one was telling me I couldn't do it. Plus, I had the backing of the clinic agency staff and the volunteer physicians I was working for. They were all part of the power elite in the state: white male Southern Evangelical Protestant Christians. I thought I was protected.

———————

Nurse practitioners are an American invention, and specifically they are an invention of the American West. The nurse practitioner role was started by a Colorado nurse in the mid-1960s during President Johnson's War on Poverty, when Medicaid and Medicare were established to extend health care to the poor and elderly. Even before this expansion of health care, there was a shortage of primary care physicians. At the same time there were many seasoned, capable nurses who were already providing basic health care to poor and underserved populations. A nurse-physician team developed the nurse practitioner role, adding additional course work and clinical training for nurses. With this, states began allowing nurse practitioners to diagnose and treat patients, including prescribing medications for common health problems.

Not surprisingly, the emergence of the nurse practitioner role met with the most resistance in states with higher physician-to-population ratios, and in states with more powerful and politically conservative physician lobbying groups. The nurse practitioner role was protested within both the medical and nursing establishments. Physicians didn't want nurses taking jobs from them, and nurses didn't want other nurses having a more direct treatment role—more power and prestige—than they did. But the role caught on and spread throughout the country. Nurse practitioners didn't get firmly established in Virginia until the mid-1980s, when I completed my training.

Why nursing? I often asked myself, and people continued to ask me even after I became a nurse practitioner. It was as if any sane, intelligent, modern woman could not want to be a nurse. I had stumbled into nursing while a master's student at Harvard University, studying medical ethics and taking courses in the School of Public Health. I was gravitating toward a public health degree, but was advised by one of my professors to go to either medical or nursing school first in order to get direct health care experience. I didn't like the approach of mainstream medicine, but also had a negative stereotype of nursing. The only nurses I knew worked in my rural family doctor's office. They were stout, dull-witted, and wore silly starched white caps, overly tight white polyester uniforms, and white support stockings that swished as their fleshy thighs rubbed together. But in graduate school at Harvard I sprained my ankle, and went to the student health clinic. I was seen by a kind and competent provider who spent time explaining what I should do to help my ankle recover. I was impressed and thought she was the best doctor I'd ever seen. Then she told me she was a nurse practitioner and explained what that was. My negative stereotype of nurses was challenged.

When I started work at the CrossOver Clinic in Richmond, I didn't understand the politics or differences between states in terms of nurse practitioner practice. Since the start of the nurse practitioner role, Virginia has consistently ranked at the bottom, along with Georgia and South Carolina, in terms of a favorable climate for nurse practitioners. These Old South states have powerful, deeply entrenched networks of traditional medical societies, like the one I had recently met with. Many of the Southern states have high ratios of physicians to the general population, yet have the worst poverty and shortest life spans of any region in the United States. These facts were not taught or discussed in my nursing school. But I was about to get a direct lesson in health care politics: a lesson that would alter my life and career.

I still vividly remember the day. It was October 13, 1988, a busy Tuesday morning, and I was seeing patients, working alone—it wasn't a day for the students to be with me. I noticed an older man walk in the clinic door. He was frumpily but professionally dressed in an ill-fitting dark-brown suit, and was balding, with oily wisps of faded red hair combed back. I thought at first he was a drug company representative, since occasionally they would drop off free samples of high-priced medications we couldn't afford to keep our patients on. He pulled out a business card and handed it to me.

"I'm doing an investigation of a complaint made to the Virginia Health Regulatory Board about your practice."

"Oh. Are you here about the dog?" I asked, thinking someone had reported me for treating Scruffy.

"What dog?" He looked at me askance. "I'm here for the Boards of Medicine and Nursing to investigate a complaint about your practice."

I was stunned. My mind raced through worst-case scenarios: had I killed a patient? The only medical mistake I was aware of having made was when I'd given the patient penicillin when he was allergic to it. Then I remembered my recent talk at the medical society meeting, and my sense of foreboding while there. I swallowed hard.

"I'm doing an investigation of complaints made about the scope of your practice, especially as it pertains to the dispensing of medications." He sounded as if he had rehearsed this line many times, alone, in front of the mirror.

"Dispensing medications?" I asked. I went on to explain how I was handling medications. I was doing what our volunteer doctors had done for years: either giving patients prepackaged sample medications from drug reps, or dispensing less-expensive bulk medicines in Ziploc plastic bags, with a white stick-on label with the patient's name, name of the medicine, and instructions for taking the medicine. None of my patients had the money or health insurance to fill prescriptions. I had a written protocol for diagnosing and treating a variety of common injuries and illnesses that Cullen had reviewed and signed for me. That's what the law in Virginia stipulated at the time in terms of practice requirements for nurse practitioners, or so I thought.

I shooed the patients out and closed the clinic for the rest of the day. After the Health Regulatory Board inspector had finished looking through charts, examining the medication cabinet, and asking me many questions, he said, "You'll be hearing from us sometime soon. It's hard to predict how long the investigation will take, but if I have any more questions, I'll call you."

I was confused. "So, do I need to do anything differently or close the clinic?"

"No, not at this point, but again, I don't make those decisions, my supervisor does. He'll let you know."

The most immediate threat of the investigation was the potential loss of my license. My salary supported my family. Charles was still in seminary and I was paying for child care for Jonathan. I knew most people would automatically assume I'd done something wrong, that I was either incompetent or immoral. My professional reputation was at stake. The investigation dragged on. I lost sleep and weight worrying about it. I had to stop nursing Jonathan because I lost too much weight. I kept working at the clinic, although in reduced capacity, and not dispensing any medications. Charles and I got in more verbal fights. He kept telling me Satan was testing me and I needed to maintain a sweet and resolute Christian outlook. But I increasingly believed in righteous indignation, including toward my husband.

The clinic board of directors responded to the investigation by enlisting the help of a volunteer lawyer who talked with the lawyers at the Health Regulatory Board. I was told nurse practitioners' scope of practice was a gray area of Virginia law. The Board of Medicine was concerned that a nurse practitioner was staffing the clinic alone, and they didn't want to establish precedence. I was the camel's nose poking in their medical tent. I didn't think of hiring my own lawyer, and I couldn't have afforded one anyway.

In mid-December I was called in for a meeting with a State Attorney General's office senior lawyer to discuss my role at the clinic. He was advising the Health Regulatory Board on my case. I did not wear Laura Ashley. Instead, I wore navy-blue pants and an off-white hand-knit sweater jacket. I went for professional but comfortable in my look since I had a bad cold I couldn't get rid of. I ditched the pearls; I was no longer feeling demure and pious.

The Attorney General's offices were in a building downtown, across the street from the bright white dome of the State Capitol Building, next door to the even-whiter Saint Paul's Episcopal Church, and a few blocks downhill from the dove-gray White House of the Confederacy. I entered the waiting room, a small, carpeted room with only a few chairs, and a stern, matronly secretary sitting at a desk in the corner and wearing heavy dictation headphones. She glanced up at me over the rims of her wire reading glasses as she typed on a purring electric typewriter.

"Have a seat. He'll be with you in a few minutes," she said loudly, without pausing her typing or taking off her headphones.

I sat down. My nose started running and I realized I'd forgotten to bring tissues. Also, sometimes when I got angry I cried. That really frustrated me and I had tried all sorts of tricks to keep myself from this sort of crying. I wasn't always successful, so I needed to be prepared.

There were no boxes of tissues in the waiting room. The secretary sighed loudly and whipped off her headphones when I asked where the women's restroom was.

"Down the hall to your right. Don't be long." She glared at me as she put her headphones back on and resumed her typing.

When I returned from the restroom, the secretary stood up, opened the lawyer's door barely wide enough for me to enter, and said, "He's waiting. Go in and have a seat." I walked in as she quickly closed the heavy door behind me.

I could barely see as I looked around for the chair I was supposed to sit in. The room was dark: dark wood bookshelves and dark-green walls and dark-green thick-piled carpeting. The only light in the room was from a small green-glass-shaded brass lamp on the lawyer's desk. His pinstripe-suited arms lay in the middle of the small pool of light. He was writing with a heavy fountain pen on a yellow legal pad. *So lawyers really do use those*, I thought.

"Good morning," he said as he introduced himself, halfway standing up and offering his hand across the desk. He was tall, blond, middle-aged, trim, and muscular. His firm, jerking handshake hurt.

"Just need to finish a thought here." He sat down and continued writing, as I sat on a stiff-backed chair facing him. Next to my chair was a small coffee table with a chess set on top. I was concentrating on getting an initial read of the man, gauging how I should act. My stomach growled loudly. I'd been too nervous that morning to eat breakfast.

"Excuse me," I said, discreetly rubbing my stomach, while gazing down at the chess set. He continued writing and didn't seem to hear me.

I stared at the chess set, noticing it was bigger than usual. The figures were about three inches high. In addition to their size, they looked odd. As I leaned over to look more closely, I realized the chess pieces were Union and Confederate soldiers. They were set up as if he were in the midst of a game with an invisible opponent. Abraham Lincoln and Jefferson Davis were kings, Varina Davis and Mary Todd Lincoln were queens, Generals Ulysses Grant and Robert E. Lee were bishops, and generic white drummers were pawns. I had grown up amidst Civil War ghosts and the KKK. I knew there were people in the South who were still into the Civil War, but I had no idea it included chess.

"Do you play chess?" he asked me suddenly, putting down his pen, folding his hands together with elbows on the desk, leaning toward me.

I briefly wondered if my answer would determine my fate in the investigation. I thought of bluffing and saying yes, since I thought that was the correct answer. But things were so odd in this office that if I said yes, perhaps he would challenge me to finish the game.

"No, not really. I think I learned years ago." Sort of the truth. I had learned the names of the chess pieces as a child, but I had been into physically active games like volleyball and tetherball. I was the summer camp tetherball champion at age ten. Even though I was petite, I was quite good at bobbling the ball and confusing my opponent. That wasn't going to help me now.

I coughed. Really coughed and couldn't stop coughing, covering my mouth and averting my face. I reached for the tissues in my pocket. "Excuse me," I said between coughs, "I've had a nasty cold I can't seem to shake."

"Well, you're a nurse aren't you? You should know how to take better care of yourself!" he said, chuckling, waving his hands over his head as if he'd said something clever.

I felt my face flush with rage. It was as if he had reached over and patted me on the head. I glanced at him, then down at the strange chess set. I thought of standing up and retreating from his office. I didn't. Instead, his voice became background noise, like the adults in the Peanuts cartoon. I suppressed my anger because I had been doing that and it was becoming second nature. I wondered if it was like the warnings I'd had as a child to not cross my eyes or they'd get stuck: was I getting stuck in dissembling mode?

At the end of the meeting he told me that our clinic filled a need for a group of people "who, God knows, no one wants to work with," and that his office would do all it could to work out a solution to the legal questions about my practice.

———————

There were large gaps of time of not hearing anything about the investigation, but I was always aware that it was ongoing, unresolved, like a noose dangling above my head. I felt powerless. I talked with some of my former nursing professors who were active in professional nursing organizations in the state. They didn't offer much in the way of assistance; they just confirmed that I had run into a major power play with the medical establishment and said,

"Good luck with that and way to go—you're a pioneer." I stopped talking to them and vowed never to become a nursing professor. I was still too young to be cautious of the vows I took.

The Health Regulatory Board closed the clinic for two weeks in April, right before Jonathan's first birthday, pending the outcome of a Medical Board meeting. They allowed us to reopen with changed rules, mainly that I was required to phone in all medications to the nearby Safeway pharmacy, at a huge cost increase to the clinic. I was disgusted. The Medical and Nursing Boards kept the investigation on me open for sixteen months, waiting for further complaints from area physicians, waiting for me to mess up, waiting for me to make a false move.

All of this fueled my ambivalence for the role of nursing. I wanted to be left alone to do what I knew I could do well: provide basic cost-effective health care to a marginalized population. But now I realized that safety net health care in our country was only tolerated when it was contained as charity care, volunteer-type health care that made the volunteers and the agency behind the care feel good about their generosity. It wasn't tolerated when charity care challenged the status quo. And nurses were only tolerated when they were subservient. These were rules to a game I didn't want to play.

CHAPTER SEVEN

Death List

THE FIRST ONE WAS a forty-eight-year-old white man who died on Christmas Day, 1986: suicide by gun. The next one died on my birthday the following June. And then another suicide, this time a twenty-eight-year-old white man who hung himself in an abandoned warehouse down by the river.

I had a list of twenty-two names of Street Center Clinic patients who had died, their birth dates and death dates, and causes of death. It was titled "Death List," and spanned the three years I had worked at the Street Center. These were only the confirmed deaths. The list included twenty men and two women; both women had been stabbed to death. Four suicides, three heart attacks, five liver failures, three died of AIDS, two froze to death, one man—Jake—

drowned in the James River, and one man was buried alive by coal while he slept in a train car. Another was a forty-six-year-old patient who lived in the old Capitol Hotel downtown. He died alone in his room—cause of death unknown. The hotel manager found his body two weeks later, alerted by hotel residents who noticed a worse-than-usual smell coming from his end of the hallway. Reading through the list, I descended into self-pity, my eyes beginning to tear—I wondered how long it would take anyone to find me if I died of hypothermia in this empty house I was lying in, alone.

Larry, the head of Freedom House, had started the Death List and I began helping him, since I often got hospital reports with the cause of death of our patients. We kept the list as a testament to the injustice of homelessness and poverty, a testament to our anger, our righteous indignation—that's what we would have said then if you had asked us why we kept the list. I also kept the list from a detached scientific perspective, thinking I could document the mortality rate of the patients I was seeing, especially the rising death rate from AIDS, and then publish a journal article based on it. I wondered who would really care if the homeless led lives that were "solitary, poor, nasty, brutish, and short," as Hobbes wrote of uncivilized, ungoverned populations. I did hope that some people cared.

It was the early morning of a weekday at the beginning of April 1989. I was lying in bed—alone with the death list—pondering insanity. Wondering what it must feel like. Wondering if it was catching—if it was hereditary.

It had been a year since the Health Regulatory Board closed CrossOver Clinic for several weeks. They were still monitoring my practice as a nurse practitioner, but this was a fact I barely noticed anymore. I now had bigger problems in my life.

When I tried to reflect back on the past year of my life, it appeared to me as a cubist painting: disruptive, dissociative, disconnected, disjointed, swirling around from different perspectives, with past, present, and future melding together. Like a cubist painting, it took stepping back a considerable distance to be able to see what it was all about.

I lay in bed in a pink-walled room, in a town house in Richmond, alone. I had left my husband. Charles had insisted on keeping Jonathan in their seminary apartment across town. Perhaps it was selfish, but I had agreed, thankful for time alone to figure out my life, thankful for space to breathe. I did not want to drag Jonathan down with me into the murky depths that had become my life. I was in survival mode and handed Jon up into a lifeboat as my own ship floundered. And I knew that he was well loved, well cared for by his father.

The furnace in my rented house was dead. It was cold inside. I heard a garbage truck emptying trash cans in the alley behind the town house. I stared at the white ceiling, with streaks of pink sun and scintillating gray shadows from the new leaves on the trees in the backyard. Pinioned by thick layers of blankets, quilts, and piles of books, I was in the state of being cold beyond shivering. I looked at a notebook lying open beside me on the bed. Names were written on a page. Some were typed and others were in my handwriting: Death List.

The day before, I had been at Lee's graveside funeral at Oakwood Cemetery. I had added Lee's name and cause of death to the Death List. This was the same day that Larry told me a young volunteer at Freedom House had hung himself—his roommate found him dead in the middle of their living room in a run-down rental house in Jackson Ward. Should I add his name to the Death List, or start a separate one for the people who were supposed to be helping the homeless?

How do you work with this sort of material every day, keeping lists of dead people, picking maggots out of wounds, being named as next of kin to people dying alone of AIDS, and not get bitter, angry, resentful at the world, at the people you are ostensibly trying to help, and angry at yourself for caring and for even being there?

It felt like a vortex drawing me into a cold, dark, viperous pit. I concentrated on trying to discern where the edge of the abyss was for me, so that I could peer over the edge or even explore the upper reaches. Some of the attraction of going down was not being sure I'd ever come back up again. But I didn't want to become part of the Death List. Lying in bed in the pink-walled room in a town house that was not mine, I yearned for sanity, for security, for home.

Home had always been my parents' house, nestled in the old-oak forest at Camp Hanover. Camp was my touchstone, my Arcadia. From the time I could write, I wandered through the woods writing haiku. One haiku I wrote when I was nine: "Into the forest, hopelessly and helplessly, the hurt cricket limps." Sunday school, summer camp vespers, and my parents all taught me compassion for God's creatures. I saved pennies for starving African children.

I had a hard time getting to sleep when I was a child. I worried about the starving children, the hurt crickets, and the bullets of the world. I worried about my father's angry, capricious outbursts. My older sister Martha, with whom I shared a bedroom, would tell me a bedtime story. The basic plot was that my best friend, Susie, and I were picking daisies beside the railroad tracks when Susie got hit by a train: thump! There was Susie in pieces all over the place. In the story I'd say with a heavy lisp, "Susie! Pull yourself together again and come on home!" Susie did. It was an exciting and reassuring story. Bad things could happen— death, dismemberment, starvation, and angry explosions. But unlike Humpty Dumpty, things could magically be put together again. I had been taught that prayer was like that.

Now, twenty-eight years old, lying in my pink-walled bedroom with insomnia plaguing me again, I kept saying to myself, "Pull yourself together again." The storytelling magic wasn't working. Prayer wasn't working.

Before the dislocation, I had been living within the clearly defined roles of Southern Christian white women: a sort of nurse-missionary to those suffering from inner-city poverty and homelessness, a dutiful daughter, a wife, and a mother. Religion surrounded me like the glass dome of a snow globe. My husband was a soon-to-be Presbyterian minister, my father was a Presbyterian minister, my maternal grandfather had been a missionary to Japan, and before nursing school I had gone to seminary to study medical ethics. There were so many other ministers in my family I had lost count of them all. And now I worked for an evangelical Christian organization with ties to the Moral Majority. I knew what was expected of me within all of these roles; there was a sense of safety in living within rigid expectations. My life was on display, an example of righteous living. Even when turned upside down and gently shaken, my snow globe of a life was beautiful, idyllic, a Southern Norman Rockwell scene. But as if I had been holding my breath underwater for too long, I began to feel suffocated within the confines of my outward identities, especially those of wife and white Christian Southerner. Breaking out of it to breathe, as I was now doing, meant shattering the snow globe. I knew my life could not be put back together in the same way again.

Charles told me that one of his more conservative seminary friends confided to him that he viewed my work with the homeless as casting pearls before swine. Charles said he wondered the same thing sometimes. I had to get him to explain this Biblical reference and, when he did, I was incredulous that anyone, and especially my own husband, would think that providing health care to homeless people was a waste of time and effort.

I felt increasingly suffocated by religion at home and at work. The federal McKinney-funded Health Care for the Homeless grant we had gotten in January had so far only meant more work for me. While the grant funded another nurse and a full-time physician for our clinic, people didn't seem to want the jobs. Finally in October we had hired a full-time nurse, Myrna McLaughlin.

Myrna was in her late forties, married, with four grown children. She was a no-nonsense, irritable sort of nurse, squat and sturdy, with short curly blonde hair and a smile that was more like a dash, cutting straight across her face. She was an energetic, conservative, fundamentalist Christian, who called herself a freelance missionary: going anywhere in the world to help out where the need was greatest. She went to the same evangelical Presbyterian church that Buddy and Cullen went to—a church Charles and I had gone to a few times—where people spoke in tongues during the services. Speaking in tongues was something Charles found comfortable and participated in, but I did not: I found it bizarre, like a room full of buzzing, lunatic hornets. Myrna was increasingly grating and officious as I got to know her. She had first volunteered with CrossOver Clinic, and then at the beginning of October began as the full-time clinic nurse and volunteer coordinator. We also hired a front-desk person for the clinic, Joyce Jones, a quiet, shy, sweet, young Mennonite who had been a Freedom House volunteer.

We didn't get the federal Health Care for the Homeless grant directly. The Daily Planet received the grant, provided substance-abuse services, and subcontracted with CrossOver Clinic to provide medical and dental care. I suppose that since Shelia and The Planet staff members had mainly been working with me over the past two years and I had written the health portion of the grant proposal, they were comfortable with the federal subcontract. They knew I was low-key about the religious aspects of the clinic. Beginning in January, when we first started to receive the Health Care for the Homeless federal funding, I changed the format and tone of my monthly clinic reports, since they now went to Shelia and to the federal government workers and not just to the CrossOver board. The reports no longer had any Christian references or tone.

In November, George H. W. Bush was elected president, continuing a conservative Republican streak of leadership in the country. Buddy and the CrossOver board members had all voted for him and were ecstatic at his victory. President Bush entered with his "Thousand Points of Light" campaign speech, "I have spoken of a thousand points of lights, of all the community organizations that are spread like stars throughout the nation," and upholding the death penalty and opposing abortion. He began a campaign attempting to blur the separation of church and state.

The principle of the separation of church and state had its founding in the United States in 1786 less than a mile from the Street Center, at the Virginia General Assembly, when they voted in favor of Thomas Jefferson's Virginia Statute for Religious Freedom. This statute was the forerunner of our country's First Amendment protections of religious freedom. Part of Jefferson's statute stipulated that no person could be compelled to attend any church or to support it with taxation. As a consequence, throughout the history of the United States, churches and faith-based organizations generally avoided accepting federal grant monies because they wanted to maintain the "right to discriminate" in hiring practices: accepting federal grants meant they had to follow federal regulations on fair hiring and not to discriminate based on religious affiliation.

I knew all of this at the time, but it had not yet registered to me that there could be a problem with Cross-Over Clinic accepting a subcontract of a federal grant. The national Health Care for the Homeless Program seemed to be a perfect fit with what our clinic was doing, and for what I envisioned our clinic doing more of in the future. I also wasn't in charge of hiring—Buddy and Cullen and the CrossOver board of directors were.

The CrossOver board of directors was composed entirely of white men, doctors, dentists, and ministers. All of CrossOver Clinic's staff and volunteers were white, and the only females were Myrna, Joyce, and myself. I pointed out the lack of gender and racial diversity to the board of directors. Buddy said they'd pray about it, and then said he knew I was busy with the clinic and with Jonathan, so I didn't need to come to the board meetings anymore.

Myrna and Joyce were both sturdy women who wore conservative clothing and no makeup. Joyce was a kind young woman, several years younger than I was, and had a quiet, nonjudgmental Christian faith. She and I became friends of a sort, although it was difficult since she and her husband, Gerald, lived in voluntary poverty in a hellhole of a basement apartment in a falling-down house in Jackson Ward. I didn't like visiting her there since it was dark, dank, and depressing.

With full-time help at the Street Center Clinic that fall, I was freed up to start doing more of the outreach stipulated in the Health Care for the Homeless grant—outreach that I had written into that part of the grant. I established an expanded satellite clinic at the nearby emergency shelter for women and children, setting up a small consulting room in a spare office in the shelter. I also decided to take more science courses in preparation for either medical school or for a doctorate in public health. I felt I had reached the end of the line with nursing—at least with what our society allowed nursing to be.

Buddy started to spend more time at the Street Center Clinic to "spread the Gospel." At the Street Center Clinic I felt watched and judged by Buddy whenever he was there, as well as by Myrna, who had a bossy way about her. She reminded me of the worst of my nursing school instructors. Buddy sat in the clinic waiting room, asked patients if they "knew and loved the Lord," and offered to pray with them for healing. If they agreed, he'd place his hand on their head, bow his head, close his eyes, and launch into a loud, long prayer right in the middle of the waiting room. Buddy also asked me for detailed information on each patient I was seeing, especially if there was a pregnancy or HIV test involved. I wanted to tell him it wasn't any of his business and that this violated patient privacy, but he was my boss and I needed the job. So I answered evasively and did more outreach on the streets and in emergency shelters where Buddy didn't follow me. I felt as if the clinic—my clinic—that I had started and run for the past two years was being taken over by Buddy and changed for the worse. I wondered how much of his increased presence at the clinic was precipitated by the Health Regulatory Board investigation. The investigation had made Buddy and the board more determined to find and hire a full-time physician for the clinic, and by that fall they had finally found their man—a white man, of course.

Dan Jannuzzi was a family physician, born and raised in eastern Virginia, who had trained at Eastern Virginia Medical School and who now worked in a small family practice in Baltimore, where he lived with his wife and two small children. He and his wife were devout conservative Christians. His wife saw the advertisement for the CrossOver job in a medical journal and encouraged Dan to apply. They drove down to Richmond to tour the clinic and interview with Cullen and Buddy and the board. I met Dan briefly when he toured the clinic. Short, pudgy, baby-faced, and grinning, he seemed nervous but nice. I wasn't included in the interview process. Dan was the only physician to inquire about the job. He accepted their offer and would start full-time in January. I was ready to hand over the clinic to him and to Myrna, and hoped to be left alone to do the medical outreach where I could continue to practice the way I wanted to. First, though, I needed a stable home.

———

Home. Where was home now? Home wasn't my childhood home in the woods of camp; it wasn't the dark, crumbling, stucco-walled seminary apartment I shared with my husband and young son. Where was it? I had never lived alone. In college and graduate school I had always had roommates. I was afraid of being alone; I yearned to be alone.

For the last few weeks of January I lived in a spare bedroom at Sheila's house in the Fan District which she shared with her teenage daughter and her husband, Kent Willis, who was about to be named the executive director of the American Civil Liberties Union of Virginia. I remember my first night at Sheila's house. I was lying in bed reading when Sheila knocked on my door, came in, and sat down on a chair beside my bed.

Leaning over with her elbows on her knees and her hands clasped together she asked, "How are you doing, Jo?"

"Okay. Kind of sad but I'm hanging in there. Thanks for letting me stay here until I find a place."

She paused, then said, "Jo, there's some things I want to talk to you about."

I froze. She sounded serious and I was afraid of what she wanted to talk about. Maybe I couldn't stay here after all. I wasn't sure where I'd go. I couldn't afford a hotel, not even a cheap one. And I couldn't live with my parents, who were both pressuring me to stay with Charles.

"All right," I managed to murmur.

She reminded me that her background was women's rights issues. I knew that she had started the Women's Advocacy Program and the Battered Women's Project at the Richmond YWCA. Sheila knew from previous conversations with me that Charles was not abusive. In some ways I had thought it would be easier for me to deal with it all if he was. I would feel more justified in leaving him. But if he had been abusive, I wouldn't have left Jonathan with him. I wasn't sure I was capable of being a full-time single mother at that point. I was feeling overwhelmed just trying to take care of myself.

"I think you need to get a good female lawyer to talk with about your situation. Not having Jonathan with you could mean Charles might charge you with abandonment and try to get sole custody. Would you be okay with that?"

An icy chill ran through my body.

"No! I hadn't thought of that. I want joint custody—I want Jonathan in my life."

"Well then, you have to be careful how you do things. I'll give you the names and phone numbers of some good lawyers I know who specialize in family law. They've got experience in this sort of thing and are smart feminists. You know Virginia has some crazy laws. With your husband a preacher, the courts would likely side with him in a custody dispute. Now get some sleep."

She gave me a quick hug and left, closing the door behind her. *Sleep*, I thought: *not likely*.

Eleven years my senior, I viewed Sheila as the older, wiser sister I wished I had. I did have two older sisters, but neither was much help. When I had tried to talk to my sister Martha about my separation from Charles, she had gotten quiet on the phone, then said, "I'll add you to our church prayer group list." Martha had married a preacher. My other sister, Jacque, was a back-to-nature earth mom who had been homeschooling her three children on a remote mountaintop in West Virginia. Jacque was married to a missionary's son.

Similar to how I had felt after Sheila rescued me from the angry outburst from Louie, I was wary of Sheila but grateful for her help. This was combined with a heightened sense of my own incompetence. I looked up to her as a role model and marveled at how smart and competent she was. I observed her with her husband and teenage daughter and was envious of the supportive, intellectual, and socially progressive home life she had. I wanted something similar. My own life seemed so far from my ideal.

The more difficult person for me to think about was Jonathan. I had to admit that Charles was the best primary parent for Jonathan in many ways—at least for now. But would I have felt this way if Jonathan had been my daughter instead of my son? I thought a son needed his father. But maybe that was convenient thinking, justifying to myself the selfishness I felt in wanting time alone, time off from the claustrophobic roles of Christian wife, mother, and nurse. I thought about these things in an endless loop all that night, then showered, dressed, and went to work doing street outreach the next day.

I talked with one of the female lawyers that Sheila referred me to. I couldn't afford her in-person consulting fees, so I only talked with her briefly on the phone. Her main advice was to try to work it out with Charles to have joint custody of Jonathan. I tried to keep things amicable with Charles. I didn't hate him, I just couldn't live with him, and I didn't want a future with him.

In early February I sublet an old town house from Ed, The Daily Planet substance-abuse counselor. He had just divorced and was downsizing to a small apartment. The town house was in the Fan District in the core of Richmond, a hipper place than any I had ever lived. I needed to be alone to sort some things out. Jonathan stayed with Charles in the seminary apartment. I had Jonathan with me in my town house on weekends and some evenings during the week. Jonathan seemed to be adapting to the separation fairly well, or at least that is what I told myself.

I remember my life's timeline by the books I read, their covers, the way they looked on my bookshelves, the way they smelled, what they spoke to me about. This period of my life was bookmarked by Joseph Campbell's *The Power of Myth,* the book version of the documentary interview of Campbell by Bill Moyers. My copy smelled musty, as it had been stored in my parents' spare bedroom. In my journal I wrote down ideas and quotes as I read through the book—grand, passionate, quixotic phrases such as, "The conquest of fear yields the courage of life."

As if living within a prolonged aura of a seizure, my life was a phantasmagoria of disconnected scenes, ideas, and yearnings. For months after moving out of the seminary apartment, I still drove across town to get gas at the same gas station. I was in a haze and afraid I wouldn't know how to pump gas at a new station. Everything in my life became confusing, except when I followed an instinctive trail of intensive reading: Tillie Olsen's *Silences,* Kate Chopin's *The Awakening*, and Charlotte Perkins Gilman's *The Yellow Wallpaper*. This, at least, was a part of my life that made sense: a feminist awakening. But it was also frightening, since in most of these stories the women who defied traditional female roles became social outcasts, and then either went insane or killed themselves. I wasn't sure which option was best.

The day I lay in bed in my pink-walled room with the Death List, I knew I was depressed. I had been seeing a therapist ever since separating from my husband. I asked my therapist for a trial of antidepressants. When he declined and my depression deepened, I called and asked him to admit me to a psych unit. I thought I could even deal with a unit like the one Lee had been locked up in. I wanted a rest cure. He told me my insurance wouldn't pay for it, and besides, it wouldn't help: depression was something I just had to live through. My previous route of Christian prayer to deal with the pain was no longer working—I was no longer sure it had ever worked. So I turned to books for answers, to see what it meant to be burned out on work and on life.

I discovered that professional burnout is a term that comes from Graham Greene's novel *A Burnt-Out Case*. In his book a burnt-out case refers to a leprosy patient who has been cured of leprosy but who has such psychological and physical scars that he is unable to reenter normal life. Greene also deals with the issue of a "leprophil": a person who is attracted to the suffering of lepers—who loves suffering and poverty and illness, a form of *schadenfreude*. The leprophil makes for a bad nurse and ends up joining the patients. The leprophil nurse doesn't take the necessary sanitary precautions to avoid catching leprosy and becomes a leper herself. All of the nurses in Greene's novel were nuns who wore traditional white habits, so the image of purity and contamination was even stronger.

I stopped adding to the Death List. It seemed pointless, as well as depressing. Dark and festering like gangrene, I had to cut out the dead portion before it spread, before it poisoned me, before I caught homelessness. I began to question what I was doing working at the Street Center, what possible good I was doing in any of the lives that touched mine. I started working with groups of people I thought were more hopeful and, perhaps by extension—although

I hated to admit it—were more worthy: young children who were homeless along with their mothers, female victims of domestic violence, and runaway teenagers. They all seemed to be more rewarding people to work with than were chronically homeless alcoholics or schizophrenic men.

What causes homelessness? Homelessness is often portrayed as an illness, caused either by individual flaws such as substance abuse or mental illness, or by societal flaws including the lack of affordable housing, the weakness of our welfare system, and the deinstitutionalization of the chronically mentally ill. Advocates for the homeless generally emphasize societal flaws, and government agency personnel and conservative politicians emphasize individual flaws. Our country is founded on the "pull yourself up by your bootstraps" mentality, so we all inherently want to believe that people are lazy or somehow defective if they are homeless and haven't "made it" in life. Perhaps our Puritan roots are responsible for the common moral judgment placed on homeless people, and that homeless people often place on themselves.

Feeding off other deeply held American values of courage, adventure, and the frontier spirit, homelessness, especially in young people, can be romanticized in Mark Twain's Huck Finn sort of way: "I reckon I got to light out for the Territory ahead of the rest, because Aunt Sally she's going to adopt me and sivilize me, and I can't stand it. I been there before."

This version of homelessness is tolerated and even socially sanctioned for young men in search of themselves, but less so for young women.

Throughout recorded history there have been different groups of people who would now be called homeless: wandering minstrels, vagrants, skid-road (or skid-row) bums, people riding the rails, hoboes, and even people on religious quests like the Christian Crusaders. The homeless, referring in this case to immigrants, or more starkly to "the wretched refuse of your teeming shores," is included in the final couplet of Emma Lazarus's sonnet, inscribed on the Statue of Liberty: "Send these, the homeless, tempest-tossed to me, I lift my lamp beside the golden door!" In one sense, all of us, except indigenous Americans, originate from homeless stock.

In public speeches, Larry used the analogy of having a family member who was struggling more than others. Maybe he or she has a mental or physical health problem, or substance abuse—this person could become homeless without their family support system, without people lending a hand or offering a place to stay. Larry said that what caused homelessness was a combination of individual vulnerabilities and failures of the various support systems: family, health care, housing, job training. I struggled with the issue of the worthy and unworthy poor, the worthy and unworthy homeless. It was an idea that was debated in the local news; it was an idea that had been debated throughout history. There were always people who were more vulnerable through no fault of their own, and there were always people who were lazy, who would take advantage of assistance. At that time, the majority of Richmonders prided themselves on their Southern hospitality and Christian charity. Most Richmonders had not yet burned out on helping the homeless.

I asked myself why people, including myself, were drawn to working with the homeless. The Christian charity idea definitely fit a lot of the Street Center staff members with whom I worked, like Larry. It fit even for myself, at least when I first began the work. Then there was the plain humanist charity of the nonreligious, like Sheila. This was the category I now put myself in. I thought about the various staff members I knew at the Street Center, and realized that many were working out their personal issues through their professional work. Many were wounded themselves in various ways, having battled alcohol and drug addictions, or having survived childhoods of extreme poverty or abuse. Some seemed drawn to the work out of guilt for a past life or action, and were doing penance for some self-convicted crime. For a few, that crime was having grown up with plenty.

My burnout stemmed from a gap between the ideal of what I wanted to do in my work, and the reality of what I was finding to be possible. I still loved working with people who were struggling with homelessness or with being marginalized. I had already experienced the powerful hand of the medical establishment, in the Health Regulatory Board limiting my work as a nurse practitioner. I began to comprehend the enormity and interconnectedness of how messed up the entire system was, to see the limits of the health care safety net, the corrupting power and oppression of Christian zealots, and the petrifying Old South mentality I lived within.

Charles wanted me to return to him in the seminary apartment. "Forsake all others and cleave only unto me," he said to me one day, after I'd moved into the pink-walled town house and had brought Jonathan back to the seminary apartment after a visit. Charles knew I was dating again. I was more shocked by the quaint wording than by the sentiment behind it.

CHAPTER EIGHT

Catching Homelessness

THREE YEARS INTO MY work at the Richmond Street Center, at the end of the summer of 1989, my father was retiring from his job at camp. My mother was packing up my childhood home, preparing to move to their new house in Richmond at the edge of the seminary, across the street from where Charles and Jonathan lived. On my days off from work, I drove to camp to see my mother and to help with the packing. I sorted out old books, their pages full of holes from silverfish. With my fingertips I traced over pencil marks on the doorpost of my childhood bedroom, marks of my height and weight, with the dates written beside them. I lay on my back on our pink Formica kitchen countertops, and looked at the undersides of the hanging wooden cabinets. There was a trail of daisies and turtles I had drawn there while chatting on the phone with my best friend. I visited the cedar tree I had kept as a houseplant when I was ten, and then planted in the front yard when it got too big for my bedroom. Pieces of me were staying behind in the house.

Beside our front door at camp, greeting people like a black lawn jockey or a large mezuzah totem, was a carved four-foot-tall mahogany statue of an androgynous figure, curled like a question mark, bent over, with its hands over its face. It was titled *Grief*. The statue stood to the right of our door for my entire childhood. I used to rub its rounded head whenever I passed through the door—as if for luck. When people asked, my mother explained it was a graduate art school project into which she poured her grief after her fiancé's death in the WWII invasion of Normandy. When I was young and at home, sick in bed, my mother would show me the blood-splattered leather pouch containing letters her fiancé had on his body when he was killed by a German sniper. These were the sorts of things she shared with me—things I was too young to understand. No wonder I grew up seeing ghosts.

Now that I was an adult, I could sometimes talk with my mother about things that worried me. She'd start off listening well, and would ask intelligent clarifying questions. I'd become hopeful we could finally have a sustained, meaningful conversation. But then she would launch into a long story about a distant relative or someone she'd once heard of or read about in a magazine like *Women's Day*, and it was always a Sunday school sort of story with a Guiding Moral Principle. I tried to tune out these stories because they often included gruesome details about some young woman's death as a result of her sins. My mother's main story to me lately was of a lovely great-aunt who ran away to Baltimore, lived on the streets, became a prostitute, and died of syphilis.

"You look so much like her," my mother said each time she finished this story. She'd smile and touch my cheek.

"Mom, why do you always tell me that?"

"Oh honey, I just want you to be careful, that's all."

"Are you telling me to not leave Charles, not get a divorce?"

"No, I'm not saying that. I just don't want you to get hurt, but I support your decision. There's something exciting about being on your own. But your father doesn't really understand your choice. It hurts him," she replied.

My father was not supportive of how I was living my life—not so much for religious reasons, but rather for appearances. "No one in our family has ever done such a thing! I won't have a divorced daughter," he told me one day that summer.

By May I was making new friends. Life with my husband had been circumscribed by church, seminary functions, and our families, who were all religious as well. I had not maintained friendships outside of that circle, not even with female friends from childhood or college. They all lived in other parts of the country by now. So I had to make new friends. Most of my friends were coworkers at the Street Center, like Ed, the chemical-dependency counselor who wanted to be a writer. And Father Ed, a Catholic priest who volunteered to help me with grant writing for the clinic.

Father Ed was tall and cowboy handsome, with a broad smile and a deep dimple in his chin. He had an endearing, low-key rebellious streak. He was an ex-Air Force pilot.

Before moving to Richmond, he had flown reconnaissance flights over southwestern Virginia, monitoring illegal strip-mining for an environmental watchdog group. "We got shot at a lot. It's a place they're used to shooting at people they don't like," he said, with a broad smile. He lived in a monastery in the West End of Richmond. We went to movies. I made him dinner and we had the most chaste of dates. Father Ed gave me grant-writing lessons, and took me on a trip to Washington, DC to search the Foundation Center database for grants to support the clinic. Through it all, he gently prodded me to enter a Catholic retreat center for rest and reflection. I was tempted. Thomas Merton had been one of my role models when I was in college, and I'd studied Western mysticism: Saint Theresa de Avila and Saint John of the Cross, and the strange desert hermits.

Father Ed and I visited Richmond Hill, a beautiful, serene site on the highest point of Church Hill, near my former patient Lee's grave site in Oakwood Cemetery. Richmond Hill had been a cloistered nunnery where they made communion wafers. It now was being converted into a lay retreat center. As I walked through the old herb gardens, around the koi pond, all surrounded by mossy stone walls with seats built into them, it felt like a good idea to move there—but also wimpy, an easy escape, like asking to be put in a psych unit, like admitting I was crazy. I was also afraid of being converted to Catholicism. It was a seductive faith, full of glittery icons, Latin chants, and powerful rituals. But oddly, it seemed more feasible to be merely spiritually grounded and not overly zealous within Catholicism. I liked the Freedom House's Dorothy Day–liberation theology approach to Catholicism, and I contemplated conversion, but I didn't get far enough to know what conversion actually entailed.

Instead of converting or getting myself to a nunnery, I took a trip to the desert of Arizona. It was early June and there was grant money for me to attend a National Health Care for the Homeless Symposium in Scottsdale. It was my first trip to the West. It was the first trip I had ever taken alone. The conference was held in a large, luxurious hotel and conference center, wrapped around a large outdoor pool. I tried to go running but was stopped by aggressive automatic sprinklers watering the hotel's golf course. It was all a jarring juxtaposition: not just the brown desert and emerald-green watered golf courses, but also the luxurious conference hotel, housing people who were either homeless, or who worked with people who were homeless.

I stayed at the conference for the minimum time possible, rented a car, and drove north through the desert toward the Grand Canyon. I made it as far as Sedona before I had to return to Scottsdale. I could only afford the rental car for one day. The federal grant was paying for the rest of my trip and hotel stay. It was exhilarating to feel so exposed, so small amidst the powerful red rock formations and the vast sky: an alien landscape. I also felt giddy knowing I could travel on my own so far from home. When I flew back into Richmond the next day, a thunderstorm had just swept through, and the lush, green, wet vegetation was a comforting change. But it also felt cloying, claustrophobic, as if the vines were slowly wrapping themselves around my neck.

My trip to Sedona was the high point of a summer that slid downhill with increasing momentum as the long, hot days went by. My money all went to pay rent, child and spousal support, and membership to the Downtown YMCA. I was swimming every day in the indoor pool. Between two to three miles every day, back and forth, flip turns at the end so I could stay underwater, mesmerized by the rhythm of my body, by the sound and feel of the water. My wedding ring kept catching on the pool wall, so I took it off. Swimming was my Prozac. Swimming was my Catholic ritual fix.

I carried a pager for my work in the shelters. I swam so much at the downtown YMCA that I had become friends with the lifeguard. He kept my pager while I swam and he waved a kickboard underwater at the deep end of the pool whenever I got a page. I'd get out, call and confer with the social workers about whatever question they had, and arrange to stop by the emergency shelter after my swim. It was typically a child with asthma who was stable but who was running out of his or her inhaler, or a mother who wanted a refill of birth control pills. Health care through street and emergency shelter outreach was more episodic in nature, with the patients passing quickly through my life. Most of the women and children at the shelter stayed there less than a week before moving into more permanent housing. I didn't get as involved with the patients as I had when I worked full-time at the Street Center. After the intensity of Lee's final days and death, I found this new distance from my patients to be a relief.

———————

By midsummer, my marriage was clearly over and I was beginning to have conflicts at work. I had been working less at the Street Center Clinic and almost exclusively doing street and shelter outreach. But Dan and Myrna were getting busier seeing patients at the Street Center, and Dan wanted me to cover clinic there more often. In a staff meeting that July, Myrna, Buddy, and I were alone in a small conference room in a realtor's office near the Street Center. The realtor was church friends with Buddy and had let us borrow the meeting space, which was in a much nicer build-ing than the Street Center. Dan walked into the conference room. He was wearing a short-sleeved button-down shirt, tie, and rumpled khaki pants. He remained standing, pulled out a paper from his briefcase, and announced he had a written statement that he had to get out of the way before we did anything else in the meeting. He then read it out loud, addressing it specifically to me, telling me he was mad as hell and wasn't going to take it anymore.

I almost started laughing, thinking Dan was doing a nerdy riff on Peter Finch's line in the movie *Network*. But see-ing the stern looks on the faces of Myrna and Buddy, I real-ized he was serious and that they knew about Dan's letter.

After Dan finished reading the letter, he turned to me and asked, "Jo, where are you going to church these days?"

Shocked at the question, I glanced down at my hands in my lap and found myself reaching for my familiar wed-ding band. I had grown accustomed to fingering my ring like a worry stone or a rosary. I could still feel a slight indentation in my finger where it had been for so many years. I decided to answer politely, honestly, vaguely.

"Well, I've decided to take some time away from church to think about some things."

"Think about what things?"

"I don't want to get into that. Besides, what does this have to do with my CrossOver job—with this meeting?"

Then Dan, Myrna, and Buddy did a quick three-way exchange of glances and all smiled briefly, knowingly, at some secret I wasn't in on. This entire encounter felt so bizarre. I pinched the back of my hand to make sure I wasn't dreaming.

Buddy responded first. "Jo, you know CrossOver is a Christian organization with a Christian mission and Chris-tian values."

"Yes, of course."

Myrna quickly added, "We expect all CrossOver Clinic staff to be practicing, committed Christians." She folded her arms, pursed her lips, and glared at me to make sure I understood what she implied.

As I looked at her, I first wondered why she thought she had the authority to weigh in on this when her official title was volunteer coordinator. Then I realized that Myrna personified what I disliked most about nursing: how rigid, dogmatic, and sanctimonious it could be. She also represented what I disliked about Christianity. But then I thought of how tedious this all was, and how I'd rather be studying organic chemistry for a major exam I had the next morning. I knew that I could be self-righteous and rigid: I had inherited some of my father's temperament. I liked to work independently and to be in charge of things. I looked defiantly at the three people sitting across the small table from me, leaned forward, and said, "I am done with this conversation. I need to think about what you've said today. I have a patient waiting for me at the women's shelter." I walked out.

My car was parked on a side street nearby. I sat in the car for a few minutes, the windows rolled up in the summer heat, expecting to fall apart and cry, giving myself time to recover before walking the few blocks to the women's emergency shelter. I was too stunned to cry.

I wrote down a few of the key phrases I had heard from Dan, Buddy, and Myrna in the meeting. I wanted to remember their exact words because I knew I would have to talk to Sheila about the meeting and seek her advice. First, I really did have a patient to see at the shelter, and then I had to study for my exam.

The following week Buddy held a two-and-a-half-hour follow-up meeting with me to discuss concerns he had about my practice, specifically my nonjudgmental stance toward people with HIV and toward pregnant women wanting abortions. He talked of instituting clinic policies on such things. It was becoming increasingly clear to me that the clinic was no longer a place I could work. But I needed the job and was hoping to keep it until I got into either medical or public health school the following year.

At the end of August, the Reverend Judson "Buddy" Childress became the official CrossOver Clinic executive director. I had been the de facto clinic director, but that all changed when they hired Dan, who became the medical director, and I ricocheted out to become the outreach coordinator. I was no longer sure what my position there really was, since my official job description had not changed. Buddy was now overseeing general clinic operations. He refused to approve my continued outreach to shelters and on the streets, instead wanting me to do outreach to local conservative Christian churches he had connections with. He wanted to focus CrossOver on "spreading the Gospel to the working poor who have a greater potential of benefiting from it than do the homeless." The working poor, the worthy poor. It now seemed that Buddy and others on the board of directors also thought we were "throwing pearls before swine" by working with the homeless.

Hundreds of people came to my father's retirement party during Labor Day weekend. Many former campers and counselors brought their families and camped out in tents over the long weekend. My father asked me to pretend I was still happily married, and he invited my husband and even my in-laws.

It was a fun but unsettling weekend, spent playing volleyball and tetherball with old camp friends who had come from all over the country to celebrate my father's retirement. It was the end of an era. My father had started the camp and then directed it for thirty-five years. Our house at camp was empty, and being torn apart. I walked through my childhood house alone, tracing with my fingers my childhood height and weight recordings in pencil on my bedroom closet doorpost. I drove back to town to sleep in my pink-walled bedroom in my rented town house.

I had thirty dollars in my checking account at the beginning of September and had to borrow money from friends to pay rent. I found myself categorized as a single, previously married, not-yet-divorced female with no independent credit history. Even though I had made the money to pay our credit card bills, I discovered that didn't count. Clearly, I could no longer afford to rent the town house, and in fact, I could no longer afford to rent a room in the city. Relishing my solitude, I had panic attacks when I thought of having roommates. I couldn't move back with my husband, and I no longer had a house at camp to return to. And most definitely I could not live with my parents in their new home. They now lived across the street from my husband and the seminary. With retirement now a reality, my father was more unpredictable, more unhinged than usual. I kept my distance from him.

In the middle of September, Buddy called me in to his office for another meeting. I had to drive to Baltimore the next morning for medical and public health school interviews. Sheila and I had been talking about my situation at the clinic; I was keeping her updated and seeking her advice. She was angry at how religiously rigid Buddy was being, especially while taking federal health care funds through The Daily Planet. She encouraged me to take a tape recorder to the meeting, since Buddy wanted to meet with me alone to "resolve some issues."

Buddy worked out of a trailer-sized building on Broad Street. It had been a real estate company. His office was small, with cheap wood-paneled walls, framed pictures of Bible quotes, and a green vinyl winged club chair. Buddy greeted me with a handshake, then sat behind his desk. The vinyl chair squeaked loudly as I sat down, emitting a dusty, plastic smell.

"Let's begin in prayer," he said, in an expansive, booming voice.

Elbows on the desk, hands clasped together, and eyes knotted shut over bristly eyebrows, he started with a prayer calling on God to guide the meeting and bless us with wisdom. I bowed my head slightly but kept my eyes open, looking at Buddy. His folded hands obscured most of his face.

With his hands still clasped together as if going for a football pass, he raised his head and leaned toward me. "Jo, you're not the same person we hired three years ago."

Thank God for that! I thought. But I tried to choose my reply more carefully.

"Well, I am, but I think I have learned a lot and grown as a person," I replied.

Our conversation disintegrated from there, but continued for over an hour. We talked past each other over and over again on just the abortion issue. After an hour I was exhausted, and told him I had to leave and get ready for a trip—I didn't tell him what the trip was for and he didn't ask.

Buddy handed me a CrossOver envelope. He told me there was a letter inside. I stared at the gray envelope with a thin, black cross printed on the front.

"Please open it so we can go over some things together," he said.

In the typewritten letter, he wrote that I had "difficulty in submitting to authority, difficulty as a team player, difficulties with interpersonal relationships, and an improper Christian faith perspective, and conflicting priorities with medical school." He read these to me, counting off the items on his fingers.

He concluded, "Effective today I am placing you on a thirty-day leave of absence, to be spent in prayer and reflection, including thoughts on your marriage." Earlier in the meeting he had asked me about the state of my marriage, saying he had heard I was separated and headed for divorce. He told me—and he'd written in the letter—that he wanted me to change into a "proper Christian woman with a teachable and humble spirit."

As part of the mandatory thirty-day leave of absence, Buddy banned me from the CrossOver Clinic. He didn't demand my keys, but he ordered me to have no contact with any of the CrossOver staff, not even by phone. He said I was creating discord between the staff and stressing them out. This part of the letter stunned me the most. I was being thrown out of the clinic at the Street Center, the clinic I had helped start? And because I was no longer Christian enough, or humble enough?

After the meeting with Buddy, I called Sheila. She again told me to get a lawyer. I couldn't afford a lawyer, and I wasn't sure I had the energy to fight Buddy even if I had the money. Sheila told me Buddy couldn't force me to take a leave of absence for anything beyond job performance issues. She asked me if I'd had regular and documented job appraisals (which I did), and if they had all been good (which they were). She asked me if I had copies of them. "No, they're at the clinic." So, that evening, before I headed to Baltimore for my medical and public health school interviews, I went to the Street Center after the clinic was closed and all the clinic staff members were gone. I took the file folder with my job performance reviews and all of my correspondence with the CrossOver board of directors over the years. Later, Joyce told me that Myrna wanted to call the police and have them charge me with trespassing when she discovered I'd been there.

The next week I spent in consultation with Sheila and a few other people about what I should do about my job situation. I canceled outreach activities. I looked for another job working for a more reasonable agency, but one where I could still work with people who were homeless. There were several possibilities, but none where I could start work immediately. I needed a job with a steady income, and preferably one with health benefits. My physical health was good, but my mental health was fraying. I knew I needed access to a therapist and I couldn't afford one without having health insurance. That week the weather was unsettled: Hurricane Hugo was headed our way. The air outside was so saturated with moisture, it felt like I was breathing underwater. Finally, on Friday, the swirling steel-gray sky began to clear and the wind settled. Hugo had weakened and passed to the west of Richmond.

I had to move, but I had nowhere to go. Already living on the edge financially, and with my job situation uncertain, I started packing. My life and my living space were contracting. I filled packing boxes with my belongings and black garbage bags with cast-offs. The boxes were filled with the tangibles of my entire life—pleasurable, memorable—but ultimately as expendable as the cast-offs in the garbage bags. I fought the urge to toss it all in the alley for the garbage truck to take away. Only my bed remained untouched. I imagined my bed as my sailboat, my life raft. Even the bed would have to be dismantled and stored away until my life settled again, like the sediment in a calm part of the river. All of the previously trusted support structures in my life were gone. I was in free-fall.

I remembered a time when I was twelve. I was swimming in the Chickahominy River near camp. Water plants, soft and furry and slimy, were growing up from the shallow water. I panicked, feeling the plants close in around me, wrapping around my legs and pulling me down toward the muddy bottom. Then I remembered my Red Cross water safety class instructions on just this scenario, and made myself relax. I turned on my back, floating, slowly sculling with my hands toward shore. The plants changed from threatening arms to comforting, tickling, and massaging fingers.

I tried to relax into the chaos of my life. My parents were pressuring me to live with them in their new house in the city. They kept saying they were worried about me. I declined their offer, but asked if I could store my belongings in their basement until I figured out what to do. I longed to be back at camp and thought of living in a tiny log cabin on the edge of the lake. But the cabin was remote and cold, only heated by a wood stove. My friendships had suffered since I had been focusing so much of my time on work and science classes. There was no one I could ask to live with. Sheila had let me stay at her house when I first separated from Charles, back in January. I knew she would let me stay again. But that sounded too needy, so I didn't ask her.

I didn't tell anyone that I had no place to live. I tried to maintain a facade of being a strong, independent, together woman. Asking for help would destroy that: I would crumble into dust.

At the end of September, my father hired me to be a maid and dishwasher at camp for the weekend retreat groups. He had had his retirement party at the end of the summer but wouldn't officially retire until January. I cleaned the bathrooms of cabins and the main lodge. I washed dishes on the weekends, a job I had done as a teenager. There I was, back in the same place, working for the same boss—my father—washing the same dishes, knocking the leftover food off them with Greasy Jane, the recirculating bubbler, before putting them through Hobart, the hot-water sterilizer. As I stared at the bubbler, now full of pieces of spaghetti and peas, and inhaled the chlorinated steam from Hobart, I asked myself if I was any closer to breaking out of the mesmerizing hold the South had on me.

It felt familiar, regressive, and demeaning, but I needed the money and I needed a place to stay. As part of working at camp, my father agreed I could live in the Trading Post, a storage shed next to the main lodge and kitchen. The Trading Post was an unheated building used during the summer months for campers to get food for hikes or cookouts. The rest of the year it was closed up and used for overflow storage for large bales of toilet paper, paper towels, and white plastic tubs of bright pink dishwashing fluid. It was next to the large walk-in refrigerator and freezer unit, as well as the trash and recycling bins. I felt I had no other option. All of my belongings had been packed up and stored in the basement of my parents' house. I felt stripped of most of the things that gave me identity: work, husband, child, faith, home, and possessions. I only had a few books, spiral-bound notebooks full of journal writing, and some clothes with me. I also had my car, a small station wagon with Jonathan's car seat strapped in the back.

The first week living in the Trading Post felt like an adventure, like camping out. Staying at camp was relaxing and quiet, and I felt safe. At night the sounds of frogs chorused around me. After the first week, the novelty of living there wore off and the frogs annoyed me. And after a month it became numbing.

I resigned from CrossOver. In my letter of resignation, I thanked the board of directors for the opportunity to work at the clinic for three and a half years, and I wished them well. "I hope CrossOver will continue to grow and to be an effective source of healing for many years to come," I wrote. I worked on the letter for a week, trying to make it truthful without sounding angry or spiteful. By the time I finished writing the final draft, I was no longer as angry. Instead, I was profoundly sad at coming to an end of my work at the Street Center in such an ignoble way.

A few days after I dropped the letter off at Buddy's office, I received a letter from him apologizing for placing me on administrative leave. He wrote, "I acted on attitudinal characteristics not becoming to a Christian. I saw some traits in you as potentially contradictory to my authority and reacted accordingly." We met in a park in Richmond to talk as we walked through the small zoo. The conversation was calm. At the end we shook hands and parted ways. I never saw him again.

I now had no job except at camp. I alternated between staying in the Trading Post and sleeping in my car on a side street in a safer part of Richmond, taking showers in the downtown YMCA after swimming. My membership there was paid through the end of the year. I was still taking physics and chemistry classes, now struggling to keep up, struggling to care about my grades or about medical or public health school. I didn't tell anyone where I was living or what I was doing. "I wash dishes and scrub toilets and sleep in a storage shed or in my car," was not something I was willing to admit to anyone. It was humiliating. I knew that if someone who wasn't a patient told me she was doing this, I would immediately wonder what was wrong with her. Plus, I would try to get away from her as fast as possible for fear I would catch her craziness—her homelessness—just by association.

By November the frost had silenced the frogs. The leaves had fallen from the trees. I lay on a foldout metal Army cot in the Trading Post. It had some rudimentary springs and an old, flattened, stained mattress on top. I propped myself up on my elbows and looked around. The Trading Post had a concrete floor stained with food and drink spills—red and purple sticky sno-cone syrup. Warped plywood shelves below a gray Formica countertop ringed the perimeter. The room was littered with chuck boxes—rectangular wooden storage boxes with rough binder-twine handles on the two short ends; these were the boxes summer groups used to pick up their food for cookouts. In one corner there was a large moldering lost-and-found pile: canteens, paperback books, a pink terry-cloth tracksuit, cutoff jeans covered in gray mud, old tennis shoes, a stretched-out purple satin bra, and many dirty socks. Looking at the pile it finally hit me: I had caught homelessness.

I was lying on the cot, in my sleeping bag, shivering. The room smelled of grape Kool-Aid and mold, mixed with an acrid tin-can smell, with an undercurrent of Pine-Sol. It felt cold—morgue-like cold, beyond hospital cold—cold as if you've already died and your body has stopped producing heat. There were periods of heavy silence. No roads or people for miles around. No airplanes passing overhead. No braying of hound dogs. No distant train whistles. It was so quiet that I could hear the whooshing ebb and flow of my blood pumping past my inner ear. Then there were periods of startling noise from outside: the motor for the room-sized walk-in refrigerator and freezer unit next door kicking on. At first it sputtered like a sleeping dragon clearing its throat, stirring in its sleep. Then it woke up with a roar, creating comforting white noise. I'd try to go to sleep while it was still running.

It didn't always work, and this was one of those nights. I tried reading. I was into Kierkegaard and Updike. Kierkegaard I was rereading for the metaphysical questions I was wrestling with in my life, especially individual responsibility and decision making. It was a book left over from one of my religion classes at Oberlin. In it I had underlined, "Life can only be understood backwards, but it must be lived forwards." I longed to be ahead, looking back. And I was reading a collection of John Updike's short stories. His description of falling in love, the great passion in "The Bulgarian Poetess," made me squirm. I kept rereading about how we fall in love with people who remind us of our first landscape, wondering who could possibly remind me of my first landscape, a landscape of ghosts and half-buried violence, covered with violets, punctuated by deep, abandoned wells. A landscape I was living in again—except I was now living within it while homeless.

Kierkegaard and Updike took too much concentration and would keep me awake. Then I tried writing in my journal. I wrote about my frustration at not being able to sleep, at not being able to at least black out for a while. I rummaged through the lost-and-found pile looking for a low-key paperback book. But they were all Harlequin romance novels I couldn't force myself to read.

Before sunrise, feeling nauseous from fatigue, I stared at a crumpled brown paper bag sitting on the floor beside me. The bag contained twenty morphine tablets. A few months before, I had had over one hundred morphine tablets. A churchwoman donated the medicine to the clinic; they were left over from her husband who had died of cancer. She thought perhaps our clinic could use the medicine for our patients, but we didn't prescribe narcotics.

I hadn't taken or sold the eighty missing tablets; I had flushed those down the toilet. But I had kept twenty of the morphine pills—more than enough to do the trick. Why had I kept them? It certainly wasn't in order to sell them, and I wasn't sure I even wanted to take them myself. I had never taken any narcotic pain meds. I had smoked pot just a few times in my teenage years and I now only drank an occasional glass or two of wine. Perhaps it was curiosity about the pills, or perhaps it was because it was strangely comforting to know I had a way out.

Lying in the Trading Post on the old Army cot, I wanted to take all of the pills now, go numb, and never wake up. It seemed easy, and I was so cold and fatigued I was not thinking clearly. It was pain medicine, after all, and I wanted the pain to go away. Specifically, I wanted to take the pills and curl up inside the walk-in freezer: to finally sleep, to submit to the cold. The thought of doing this crept up from some deep part of me. It was more of a recurrent vision than a conscious thought. It all felt so comfortable and right and peaceful. I knew it was a crazy idea, but every time the sleeping dragon sputtered awake with its engine purr, instead of white noise lulling me to sleep, it became white noise drawing me into its belly.

CHAPTER NINE

Going Under

"RELAX NOW. COUNT backwards from ten," the anesthesiologist said as he pushed amber fluid into my IV with a large syringe.

I didn't have a choice. He was forcing me to relax. I remember counting out loud to eight, and then everything went white and cold and blank. When I awoke, Dr. Danny DeVito's fat face was beaming down at me. He was short and his face was only inches from mine. His breath was hot and pungent. I coughed.

"Ah. You're waking up. Good! Good! Everything went well with the surgery. I was watching. Amazing with the laparoscope! Never seen that before. Your doctor will be around in a bit to tell you more."

I had a steamy oxygen mask over my face and my voice didn't seem to work, so I nodded feebly, groggily trying to remember how I knew Dr. Danny DeVito. I was cold. My bones were cold. The fluid running into my right arm from an IV was cold. I could feel it spreading coldness up through my arm and into my body. My floating hysteric uterus and I were cold. *Wait. Do I still have a uterus? Maybe if I count backwards from my surgery I can remember what happened. Maybe I can remember how I know Dr. Danny DeVito,* I thought, as I drifted off again.

In the South, the spirits of the place float in the vapors, lurk in the soil, enter through every pore. In the South, in the summer, amidst the fecund kudzu and the cloying damp air, life becomes exotic. In the South in the summer of my thirtieth year, my life became a freak show, a mythical monster. It had to be cut out before it destroyed me.

It was late August 1990, almost a year since my life had blown apart, since I had been lying on the Army cot in the Trading Post, contemplating the morphine pills, hearing the roar of the walk-in freezer and wanting to crawl in there and sleep. A year since I had first realized I was homeless. Not literally on the streets in the gutter homeless, but marginally and precariously housed homeless. "Precariously housed" had a certain charming ring to it, as if I had been a jittery-but-still-elegant tightrope walker for the past year and not some crumpled, broken refuse on the cement below. In any case, there was another cold winter in Richmond rolling toward me.

My life was still chaotic. No, it was more chaotic. Over the past year I had lived in seven different places—eight if you counted my car. That night in the Trading Post, when I had come close to taking all the morphine pills, had catapulted me out of the recirculating bubbler of my life, or at least partially out of it. The night had frightened me into realizing I wanted to live. I yearned to get my life back together and become a decent mother for Jonathan. I moved out of camp and lived in my car for a while. Then in December I house-sat for my parents for a month while they were in Florida. My mother asked if I planned to commit suicide at Christmas. She asked it matter-of-factly, along with asking me to forward their mail. I hadn't told her anything about my near suicide attempt, but she knew I was still depressed.

The worst place I lived that year was a subsidized low-income apartment in a cinderblock building at the edge of the West End of Richmond. It was all I could afford or qualify for on my own. It resembled a prison complex from the outside, and it felt like a prison inside. The heavy metal door of the main entrance closed with a decisive clang—just like the door in prisons, or on locked psych units. I lived there for four months, frozen in depression and limbo, not seeing a way out. Then there were four other places where I lived briefly, for several weeks each, passing through various men's apartments or houses. Most recently, and just a few months before my thirtieth birthday, I had moved into the basement of the Junior League headquarters downtown.

The prison apartment had been a nightmare. I mostly lived on bagels and coffee and an occasional vitamin pill. I lost a lot of weight, and I was already thin. The heat in the prison apartment blasted day and night and I had to keep the windows open, even in the cold of winter. I couldn't always do that, though, because people in the apartment below mine chain-smoked, and their smoke poured in through my window. I developed asthma. And migraines. Cockroaches scurried over the kitchen floors, sink, and countertops. Rats left large black droppings. I avoided going to the kitchen. Cockroaches and rats didn't scare me; they just reminded me of the realities of poverty and of what my life had become. The couple in the apartment below argued loudly and threw things, including each other, against the walls. Police came. Often. One night I awoke to gunfire, sirens and flashing red lights. I looked out my bedroom window and saw a policeman holding a rifle and crouching beside my station wagon, Jonathan's car seat silhouetted against the swirling red lights.

In this apartment from hell, I got anonymous phone messages from a woman calling me a whore. This happened every couple of weeks. The phone calls were targeted and hate-filled, an omnipotent, anonymous, evil miasma trying to suffocate me. I also thought I deserved them, since by then I was dating different men. When the phone calls came, or when the violence in the apartments around me escalated, I escaped to sleep in my car in shopping mall parking lots, or on side streets far away from this apartment. I didn't want to admit to anyone that I was afraid.

My husband had filed for divorce. He said I was leading him into the Valley of Death. In the spring he was graduating from seminary and moving farther south, to a small rural church. He was taking Jonathan with him. I tried to convince myself that it was best for my son. He needed a stable place to live, with an emotionally intact parent. At this point, I could offer neither.

Since leaving my marriage and my job, I had been trying to find a new life as a liberated, divorced, agnostic Southern woman. I was beginning to wonder if such a life in the South was possible. Besides having an unstable living situation, I now worked three part-time jobs.

I was the nurse practitioner for the women's clinic at the University of Richmond's student health clinic. All their doctors were male. University of Richmond was a conservative Baptist college, so I dealt with many female students confessing Christian guilt over their sexuality. I started them on birth control pills and wrote notes to their parents explaining the pills were for painful periods.

I also worked part-time as the nurse at the YWCA Battered Women's Shelter, staffed mostly by righteous feminists who reminded me of Sheila. Sheila had started the shelter, and she helped me get this job. Through the shelter workers, I was learning some of the complexities of intimate partner violence, such as codependency, the erosion of self-esteem, and trauma bonding: the strength of the emotional bond formed by occasional violence mixed with caring, with what passes as love. I was told I had a special affinity for the women in these situations. I didn't realize that wasn't necessarily a good thing.

My third job was at the Fan Free Clinic, a clinic modeled after the Haight-Ashbury Free Clinic, which had opened in San Francisco during 1967, the Summer of Love. I worked as a nurse practitioner in their evening clinic, mostly screening for HIV and other sexually transmitted infections. One of my coworkers, a lovely man who made an even lovelier woman, gave me lessons in how to strut correctly in high-heeled boots. He was into auras and crystals, and he gave me a large white quartz crystal to help focus my spiritual energy. And for my fourth job, I did homeless shelter outreach for the clinic.

The Fan Free Clinic had taken over the Health Care for the Homeless federal grant, and they were now running the Street Center Clinic. A CrossOver board member told me that they'd been ordered by Sheila and The Daily Planet board of directors to desist from overt religious activity as part of health care, and to maintain fair hiring and firing practices in order to keep the federal grant. The CrossOver board refused, so they lost the federal grant funding and moved to a church site across the river, where they were focusing on serving the working poor. When I heard this, I felt simultaneously detached, vindicated, and sad that it had come to that. I wondered how much disruption in health care provision there had been for some of my patients, like Louie, Sally, Harold, Bruce, and the River Rats.

Fan Free Clinic had hired a full-time doctor to work at the Street Center Clinic. She was overwhelmed by patients and kept asking me to come work with her. While I knew how it felt to be overwhelmed there, I mainly wanted to avoid the whole issue, which only made the situation worse. She was a kind and competent doctor and would have made a terrific coworker. But I couldn't explain to her the powerful revulsion I now had for the Street Center. In my mind, it was the place where my life had blown apart and gone spiraling out of control. The Street Center stood for a terrifying, disorienting, humiliating time in my life—a time I was still living through. Whenever I drove past the brick building, my palms sweated, my shoulders hunched in a defensive cringe, and I tried to avert my eyes. I wouldn't work there again. I didn't want to say why. I couldn't say why because I didn't fully understand it myself.

My part-time jobs all felt temporary. I couldn't envision myself doing any of them for very long, but I wasn't sure what my alternatives were. I needed to make enough money to support myself, as well as to support Jonathan and Charles. I was paying child support and spousal support each month. I had no health insurance and got my health care at Fan Free Clinic from one of its volunteer doctors. I took advantage of a worker's discount and got career counseling at the University of Richmond's Women's Center. They told me I should be a writer, a doctor, a public health scientist, or a cryptologist. I already knew writing didn't pay; I did not want to become a starving artist on top of being homeless. I was tired of trying to play the medical school game, and was less convinced I really wanted to be a doctor. And I had never heard of cryptology. I had started off in public health school before sidelining into nursing. I liked public health, so I decided to work toward that. But there were no schools of public health in Virginia. I'd have to go either south to North Carolina, or north to Maryland. I did not want to move any farther south, so I set my sights on Johns Hopkins in Baltimore.

The problem with working toward a new goal was that I kept losing myself. I had seen a therapist sporadically, whenever I could scrape together enough money. My therapist wanted to try hypnosis, an idea that sent me into a panic. I didn't want to lose whatever thin sliver of control I had—whatever slight hold I had on sanity, whatever glue held together the molecules of my body, of my soul. Finally, desperate to figure out what was behind my confusion and messed-up life, I agreed to try hypnosis. I don't remember much about the session, except that my therapist tried to convince me the world was a safe place. There were ambulance sirens outside his office window when he said this, but even without them, I would never believe him. Hypnosis made me fuzzy-headed for weeks. I would lapse into another realm at the most inopportune moments, including when I was working or driving or swimming. Hypnosis made me feel even more thin-skinned, porous, and blown apart: all of my molecules and energy were free-falling out into the universe.

Everything in my life, including my sanity, felt tenuous.

My part-time jobs all felt as temporary as my living situation, as temporary as my relationships.

I was having a love affair with a married doctor—I'll call him Lyon, because as far as I know I've never dated or even known a Lyon. I was trying to get beyond this affair by having brief sexual flings with whatever men I found halfway intriguing. I found them at work, I found them at the pool, and I found them while rowing on the James River. Lyon encouraged me in these sexual encounters and asked for detailed descriptions of them afterward. I tried to become what I imagined was male in sexuality: able to split off sex from feelings. As with swimming and rowing, I thought more practice would help. I was enjoying sex for the first time, but by late spring, a few months before my thirtieth birthday, sex was becoming physically painful. I joked that sex made my teeth chatter inside, not knowing how true that was. Late at night when I couldn't sleep, I imagined the pain was God's punishment for leaving my husband and for having sex with too many men.

Lyon and I met at work over the care of Lee, the black man who died of AIDS, the black man who was my next of kin. I had felt it was all meant to be. Lyon was tall, physically fit, and self-assured in an alpha-male way common to tall male doctors. He read Tom Clancy novels, flew small planes, smoked a pipe, and vacationed at Cape Hatteras with his family. When he took me out to dinner, I was entranced by his beautiful hands that trembled slightly when he held a glass—of water with a twist of lime; he was a recovering alcoholic. He was over a decade older than I. Occasionally he would tell me he loved me but that he couldn't leave his wife. He always followed this with, "Basically you could screw me." He pronounced this as a firm declaration, as if he enjoyed the risk.

When we were alone in my apartment, or in an upscale hotel room, he was sensual and slow in his lovemaking. He massaged my head, my face, my neck, my chest, sucking in air with a low moan, repeating how he wanted to be a sculptor. It started off feeling good, it was exciting. But then it became disturbing. It made me feel cold, numb, inert like clay, as if the warmth and substance of my life and soul were being sucked out of me. He palpated the veins in the bend of my arm and the vertebrae in my lower back—counting off vertebrae as he probed—"L3, L4, L5—ah—right there," exclaiming how he'd love to do a spinal tap on me, draw my cerebral fluid and then my blood.

Sex has the uncanny ability to unearth old sites of damage. When I started crying immediately after sex, with Lyon, with anyone, even with myself, it was only partially because of a growing pain in my abdomen. Sex took me to a deep, murky place, like the bottom of a pool or river. It took me to what I was really feeling. Lonely. Empty. Cheap. An object. I wasn't the type of person who should be in this situation. I wasn't supposed to be the Other Woman. I didn't see myself as the typical victim of intimate-partner violence. I didn't present myself that way to the world, to my therapist, or even to myself. I willed an outward bravado of being a strong, powerful, and independent woman. The physique I had acquired swimming and rowing strengthened the facade.

My life became a sex house of mirrors, with sex fractals splitting out into more bizarre sex realms. Lyon took photographs of me nude. I enjoyed the attention he paid to my body. He said he kept the photographs in a locked drawer in his office at work, where no one could find them. He joked about getting into swinging with me. I found the idea of sex with other couples demeaning, and figured it meant I wasn't exciting enough for him anymore, but I didn't tell him these things.

When several months went by without Lyon bringing up the swinging-sex idea, I was relieved and thought perhaps it had been only a fleeting fantasy of his. Then he had to go out of the country for six weeks on an international aid assignment in the Persian Gulf. He asked me to pick up his mail from a secret post office box he kept for receiving porn. I agreed to do it, feeling honored that he trusted me with this task and with his private mailbox key.

It was late spring when Lyon left for Saudi Arabia. I was swimming every day and had added rowing lessons to my daily routine. I enjoyed pushing my body to learn a new sport, to get stronger and leaner. Rowing also helped with balance, with my sense of where my body was in the world.

On Friday afternoon of the first week that Lyon was gone, I grabbed the key he'd given me and drove to the posh West End post office to check his mail. Inside the shiny brass box was a rolled stack of mail held together by a thick rubber band. I grabbed it and walked out quickly to avoid having a postal worker make eye contact with me.

Back at my apartment I opened the bundle. A folded piece of yellow legal paper fell out: "Jo—great photo! It worked. We've gotten a ton of responses. I've already answered the couple from Cape Fear. We'll go down there this summer when I get back—Lyon." My eyes caught on the space before he signed his name. I looked for a "love" or even an "XXOO." But that wasn't his style.

I stared at the collection of boobs and penises in the swingers' magazines now splayed on my lap. He's already made arrangements with some couple to swap partners or whatever it is they do, I thought. And where the hell is Cape Fear? But wait—what photo?

He had marked it with a medical chart red sticky tag, printed "Sign Here." I opened to the page, and there I was naked, spread belly down across a bed. My first thought was that rowing and swimming were good for my butt, followed by a choking feeling. Lyon had never told me he was planning to use a nude photo of me as a sex ad in a magazine. I looked closely at the photo, remembering the afternoon he had taken it. I'd felt sexy, powerful, desired. I checked out my head and face in the photo, anxious to see if I could be identified. Was this sort of thing illegal?

I had been trying to view all of this as feminist empowerment, as merely waking up to my sexuality after an overly repressed Southern Christian upbringing. I had told myself that it was my choice to do these things with Lyon. When I saw my naked butt in a magazine, I knew it wasn't something I chose to do, but I had no idea how to extricate myself from the relationship.

At the end of June, on my thirtieth birthday, Lyon was still in Africa. My birthday involved silk bikini underwear—black, with tiny pink rosebuds—given to me by a man I barely knew. While lying on my back in a loft in his geodesic dome amidst the odor of cooked broccoli, garlic, sweaty bodies, chlorine, and post-sex funk, I realized something was wrong.

My whole body was sore. The week before my birthday I had competed in the Chesapeake Bay Bridge Race: nearly five miles of cold, fast-moving water between Annapolis, Maryland and the eastern shore of Virginia. I was coping with life by basting my brain cells with endorphins: running, rowing, and swimming every day, but mostly swimming—at least two, sometimes three or four miles each day in the downtown YMCA. No matter how much I showered and sprayed myself with perfume, I smelled of chlorine. It made me feel deeply cleansed. There were times in the pool when I'd feel myself slowly dissolving into the water, pulled down into the dark blue depths. I relaxed into it and felt I was breathing through gills.

I had 12 percent body fat and had cut my long blonde hair into a sleek bob to make it easier to swim. For the Bay Bridge race I wore a neoprene vest, a partial wetsuit given to me by my swim coach at the YMCA. This was my first open-water swim. I knew there were aggressive male triathletes who did these races—I did laps with them in the pool and enjoyed outpacing them—but I wasn't prepared for how they started the race. I plunged into the icy gray water from the shore and was immediately pushed underwater by men clawing their way over me. I sputtered, swallowed briny bay water, then muscle memory took over and I fell into the familiar rhythm of freestyle.

Halfway through the race my hands and feet went numb. Then my arms and legs went numb. When I turned my head to the side for a breath, through foggy goggles I saw the looming concrete pillars of the bridge and the black race number written on my left bicep. I hallucinated that the bridge was a war ship and that the black number on my arm was a Nazi concentration camp number—a concentration camp I was escaping from. I briefly realized I had hypothermia and should grab onto an orange safety kayak floating nearby. Instead, I kicked harder and got through the churning center channel to warmer water. With the warmth I became lucid and finished the race.

The wet-suit vest from the bay swim had rubbed a deep abrasion in my right shoulder blade, and all of my muscles were sore from the swim a week later. But as I lay on the futon bed looking up at the dimly lit geodesic dome above me, I knew something else was causing pain. I saw from the red-lighted digital alarm clock that it was 3 a.m. My lower left abdomen throbbed and I felt waves of nausea, each wave growing stronger. I didn't want to throw up in the geodesic dome with a man I had just met. I hurriedly dressed and drove back to my apartment.

I lived alone in the basement of the Junior League headquarters, a stately old brick-and-limestone Beaux -Arts affair with black iron fencing and tall magnolia trees, located downtown, a block from the YMCA where I swam. My apartment was carved out of the old servants' (or really slaves') quarters, with an entrance off the alley, across the street from the grand Jefferson Hotel. The hotel's towers sent long shadows through my barred bedroom windows and across my bed. With its recent renovation, the Jefferson was now the plushest hotel in Richmond. I often thought about how Margaret Mitchell had stayed there while writing *Gone with the Wind*. Sometimes I put on a longer, more conservative dress, tucked a notebook in my purse, and walked around the block so the doorman at the Jefferson wouldn't see me emerging from the basement servants' quarters. I pretended I could afford to stay at the hotel; I strode in, sat in the elegant lobby, sipped coffee at a table tucked beside a potted palm, and wrote. Mostly I gazed at the red-carpeted grand staircase, envisioning a drunk and impassioned Rhett throwing Scarlett over his shoulder and taking her upstairs to the bedroom. I thought the grand staircase in the Jefferson was the most romantic place on earth—until the manager of the Battered Women's Shelter pointed out to me that, in the staircase scene, Rhett rapes his wife.

The Junior League ladies met on the main floor of the building where I lived. I saw them from the back-alley windows of my apartment. They wore tasseled Pappagallo shoes, Talbot's jackets and skirts, and strands of large pearls.

I sometimes had to walk through their main living room to visit a young couple living in the attic apartment of the building. Whenever it coincided with one of their meetings, the Junior League ladies would suddenly stop talking, stare at me, whisper to each other, and then resume their conversations. I knew the ladies had seen me going in and out of my apartment with different men. One of the men was the real estate agent who had arranged for me to rent this apartment. Like Hawthorne's Hester with her scarlet letter, I felt exposed on the town scaffold.

After my disastrous birthday night with the man in the geodesic dome, I realized I needed real health care—not just the piecemeal charity care I was getting at Fan Free Clinic. This meant I needed a job with health insurance. I was young and healthy, but I realized that a major illness or accident could ruin me financially and could send me tumbling back into homelessness. So that summer I cut back on my other jobs and took a full-time position with the Fan Free Clinic. As I waited for my health insurance to begin, I hoped whatever was inside me causing the pain wouldn't explode.

Once my health insurance became effective in early August, I went to see my gynecologist. I didn't like her—she was gruff—but she had my medical records, and I didn't want to start over with another doctor. When she finished my pelvic exam, she rolled back on her exam stool, flicked off her gloves, and said, "Okay. You can sit up now. Your left ovary is enlarged. We need to get an ultrasound. Soon."

I knew she could be pushy and prone to unnecessary testing, but I could no longer ignore the abdominal pain. It felt like a stubbed toe or an abscessed tooth—the pain throbbed with my heartbeats. I could feel it with every flip turn in the pool. And sex was getting more painful. I got the ultrasound.

My doctor delivered the ultrasound results in a voice message on my home answering machine: "You have an ovarian tumor. It's large and you need to have it removed. Call me so we can schedule surgery."

The pain in my abdomen had subsided by that time and I didn't want surgery, so I ignored my doctor's calls until she left a message informing me I had a teratoma that could be cancerous. That got my attention. I had heard of teratomas but didn't know much about them.

I pulled out my medical reference books. Teratoma, monster tumor, or deviant dermoid cyst germ cell tumor: an encapsulated cystic tumor typically lined with keratinized squamous epithelium (hardened skin), with abundant sebaceous (oil) and sweat glands, usually hair and sometimes teeth, bones, neural (nerve) tissue, and sometimes even a fetus. *Okay—gross*, I thought, but it got even stranger. Teratomas develop from genetic material contained within a single oocyte (egg) from asexual reproduction, or parthenogenesis (Greek for "virgin birth").

So the teratoma in my left ovary, the monster tumor beating in time with my own heart, was a sort of a clone of me, growing inside me? *My chimera*, I thought.

I called my doctor. She told me that it appeared I had several teeth and perhaps vestiges of an embryo in my left ovary. She recommended I have surgery within a few weeks. The tumor could rupture or it could be cancerous and spread.

Stunned, I spent time thinking about my toothed ovary, my toothed vagina: Freud's source of men's castration anxiety. Witches were thought to have toothed vaginas in the Middle Ages and were killed for them. Later I would discover that teratomas can cause limbic encephalitis—swelling of the deepest, most primitive part of the brain—complete with migraines, acute psychotic episodes, and inappropriate smiling. Freud was right: ovaries cause insanity.

Rowing and swimming were the only things keeping me sane, and I did not want surgery to interrupt them more than necessary. I found a female surgeon who at the time was the only one in Richmond able to do abdominal surgery with a laparoscope. I'd have a few small incisions below my bikini line and I could be back rowing and swimming in a few weeks. She told me she would check my tumor for cancer while I was under general anesthesia, and if it were cancerous, she'd have to take out my other ovary and my uterus.

I was more afraid of general anesthesia than I was of the surgery or even of the possibility of having cancer or of losing my fertility. I was afraid of being separated from myself, of losing control. But then I started thinking of all the other things that could go wrong during surgery, including bleeding so much I'd have to have a blood transfusion. Lee's painful death from AIDS was still fresh in my memory, and HIV was still essentially a death sentence. The blood banks had been having problems with adequately screening for HIV, so my surgeon recommended I bank my own blood.

At the blood bank one hot, humid August afternoon, the technician handed me a clipboard containing a thick sheaf of consent forms, along with an HIV questionnaire. As I began filling out the paperwork, I stumbled over the question, "How many sexual partners have you had in your lifetime?" I gazed over at the distant whitewashed wall and started counting in my head. Then I remembered I had to add the geodesic-dome man.

I looked at the blood-bank questionnaire, and wrote in my lifetime sex partner number. I hoped the technician wouldn't review the forms. "Okay. Finished. Ready to take my blood?" I held my arm out for the tourniquet. The young male technician tightened it around my arm.

I woke up in the hospital room at night with the lights dimmed, an IV still dripping in my arm. I had several blankets piled on me; I was no longer cold. My surgeon walked in briskly and pulled up a chair beside my bed. We were alone in the room. She told me the surgery had gone well, that there was no sign of cancer, so she had only removed my left ovary. I could go home the next morning. No sex or rowing or swimming for two weeks. I nodded and thanked her.

As I watched her white form walking out the door, I remembered who Dr. Danny DeVito was. Dr. DeVee was a nickname the nurses had for the OB/GYN doctor at the University of Richmond clinic where I worked. What was he doing observing my surgery?

For the following week, I was alone in my basement apartment in the bowels of the Junior League building. One morning at dawn while lying in bed, I gazed through the tops of my barred windows at the Jefferson Hotel lit by the rising sun. For the first time I noticed how ugly its muscular square towers were. I focused instead on the pale-aqua medicine bottles and the clear quartz crystal that lined my windowsill. The crystal sent prisms of sunlight dancing over my eyelet bedcover, over the star-shaped stitches in my belly where the laparoscope and instruments had been threaded through my skin.

I knew then that I was done living in servants' quarters in the shadows of the *Gone with the Wind* hotel. In order to survive, I needed to kick like hell, leave the chaos of homelessness and the murkiness of the South behind.

CHAPTER TEN

Greyhound Therapy

And the end of all our exploring
Will be to arrive where we started
And know the place for the first time.
—T. S. Eliot

I HAVE A RECURRING nightmare of working on an assembly line where faceless broken bodies move past me at increasing speed. My job is to patch them together, but I can't keep up. They remain broken—and silent—falling off the end of the conveyor belt onto a growing pile. I know the nightmare is about my work as a nurse with homeless people, work I have done for over thirty years.

The truth is that not all of the bodies on my nightmare assembly line are faceless or silent. Some have the distinct faces and voices of homeless young people with whom I have worked. Homeless young people haunt me in a way that homeless adults never have. The worst hauntings are by homeless young women, perhaps because young women are more vulnerable. Or perhaps because I have been a homeless young woman. In my dream I see my own body, mute, between the bodies of two homeless young women— between two specific young women.

———

One evening in 1996, at the homeless youth clinic in Seattle where I worked as a nurse practitioner, I looked over the medical chart of a new patient. She went by her street name—Dazzle—and she had just turned sixteen. I opened the door to find her sitting cross-legged on the exam table, undressed from the waist down, a paper sheet draped over her lower body. Dazzle was thin, olive-skinned, with black cascading wavy hair, a dark ruby-red nose piercing, and a tattoo of a red rose across her left breast, the tattoo sprouting from the top of her tight-fitting camisole. She sat hunched over, chewing her nails. With her hazel eyes she glanced up at me as I greeted her.

"It says here on your chart that you're here to get a vaginal infection checked out. Can you tell me more about what's going on?"

"Yeah. I think it's a yeast infection 'cause I've gotten 'em before. This one's so bad though it hurts to have sex. My boyfriend, he's gonna want to have sex tonight, so I was hoping you'd give me some pills to make it better faster."

When I examined her she had such a bad vaginal yeast infection that it hurt to look at, she was so raw and red. In response to my questions, Dazzle told me she lived with her boyfriend in a motel on Aurora Avenue. From what she said—and from what she didn't say—I knew he was really her pimp, and that she'd have to work that night as a prostitute.

Aurora Avenue, old Highway 99, is a long-established track for prostitutes in Seattle, lined with cheap hotels, adult sex shops, and motorcycle and gun stores. There is even an exotic meat store that sells elk, buffalo, and rattlesnake. Built on top of an old wagon trail, Aurora is a stretch of highway that keeps Seattle firmly tethered to the remnants of the Wild West. South of the city it's called Pacific Highway South. This is the stretch of road where Gary Ridgway, the Green River killer, picked up young prostitutes he would rape, strangle, and toss from his truck, covering their bodies with trash or dumping them in the nearby river. He lost count of how many he killed. When I saw Dazzle in clinic, Gary was still murdering prostitutes.

"Can I bring in someone who can talk with you about safer places to stay tonight?" I wanted Dazzle to talk with our mental health counselor without using that specific title, since it made young people think I was labeling them as crazy.

But she got increasingly agitated, said, "No, really, I'll be fine, I just need those pills to make this go away," and left. She never returned.

Her body is one of those beside mine on the nightmare conveyor belt.

A large number of our youth clinic patients worked in the sex industry as exotic dancers and prostitutes. Most came to clinic by themselves, some were brought in by their pimps, and a few young females came in with their male high school teachers who were fleeing other states on criminal sex charges. I was never sure which I found more despicable: the pimps or the teachers. The prostitutes were mostly young women, although there were also young men and transgender youth.

We called it survival sex or just plain sex work, and erred on the side of nonintervention and harm reduction, trying to keep the young people as safe as possible until they could exit "the life." This was a laudable goal and one I believed in. But in effect there were times we were supporting their lifestyle, enabling it, and becoming part of the problem. We mostly used the neutral term "sex worker" instead of "prostitute," thinking it was more politically correct, more respectful of the young people involved.

I often asked myself: Is it possible for someone to be involved in commercial sex work and have healthy self-esteem? Is there such a thing as a happy, healthy hooker? Is the character Julia Roberts plays in *Pretty Woman* based on any sort of reality, or is she just part of a twisted fairy tale? I know prostitutes who call it a profession, who say they freely choose their work. I'd like to believe them because it would make my work easier. But their statements have the off-key clang of the false bravado I know so well, having used it myself over the years. So many young prostitutes have histories of previous sexual abuse as children. Their bodies are not their own; their bodies have been stolen from them. In such situations, free choice is not possible.

I learned this early in my career from the first homeless teen I ever worked with. Dawn is the homeless girl who haunts me the most, perhaps because she was in my life the longest, or because of how our lives converged. Hers is the other body beside mine in my nightmare.

———————

It was early June 1987 in my hometown of Richmond, Virginia. This was the summer I lost my faith; this was the summer I began my own spiral into homelessness.

Dawn was fifteen when I met her. I was doing street outreach with the Richmond Street Team, which operated out of the Street Center. Dawn had been living on the streets for three months and was involved in prostitution. The Street Team's social workers and mental health counselors were trying hard to get Dawn into Oasis House, the only teen shelter in Richmond. She refused, saying she didn't want to live in a place with curfews, chores, and young bratty residents.

The Richmond Street Team was a three-year-old outreach program of the Richmond Department of Mental Health, Mental Retardation, and Substance Abuse. The Street Team consisted of six people with expertise in mental health, social services, and substance abuse. They focused on identifying homeless adults and teens with mental health and substance-abuse issues, and linking them with available services—mainly with emergency shelter beds. There were only a dozen or so publicly funded drug and alcohol inpatient beds in the city, with months-long waiting lists. None of the available outpatient drug-and-alcohol-treatment programs effectively dealt with people who had co-occurring mental health disorders. Most of our homeless patients fell into this category. The few available mental health treatment programs didn't accept patients with active substance-abuse problems. Street Team staff members did their best to connect people with whatever services they could find.

Dawn had run away from her home in a small coal-mining town in the Appalachian mountains of western Virginia. She traveled to Richmond on a one-way Greyhound bus ticket, hoping to stay with an older sister. But her sister wouldn't let her live with her, fearing Dawn would steal her boyfriend. Instead, Dawn found a group of men staying in tents on the edge of an open area near the Greyhound bus station. They let her stay with them, eat their food, and drink Wild Irish Rose in exchange for sex. Dawn was used to taking care of herself. She was used to survival sex with men. Her mother was an alcoholic and her mother's live-in boyfriend had been sexually abusing Dawn for years.

Dawn told me pieces of her story as I worked with her over the next two years. Her story was an example of Greyhound Therapy, what Alcoholic Anonymous calls the geographical cure: attempting to escape problems by moving somewhere else. The Big Book states that it doesn't work, and quotes Confucius: "Wherever you go, there you are." Especially for young people like Dawn, escaping damaging home situations made sense, but the alternatives awaiting them weren't much better.

The day I first met Dawn, she was standing with a group of young men in the parking lot of a take-out pizza place just a few blocks north of the Street Center. Dawn was big in the Matisse way: fleshy, voluptuous, exuding sexuality like an early-blooming flower having just peaked and beginning to decompose. She had a small head, short bowl-cut sandy hair, and glacier-blue eyes. Her voice was a loud baritone, out of sync with her large, sagging breasts. She was braless and wore a men's undershirt, with a faded cotton high school letter jacket and baggy torn jeans. Dawn was laughing, sneaking up behind one of the taller men, jumping up and trying to knock the baseball cap off his head in a pesky, flirtatious way.

"Hey, Dawn, I want you to meet Nurse Jo. She's the one I told you about from the Street Center Clinic." One of the Street Team counselors was trying to get Dawn's attention as she continued to jump after the man's hat. Now that she had an audience, Dawn got even more boisterous.

"Damn it all, Dawn, quit it now!" The man with the hat finally had enough. "Leave me alone before I have to hurt you!" He pushed her away.

Dawn had a look on her face like a slapped puppy, stung by his words. Then she frowned and looked down at her feet, kicking loose gravel from a muddy pothole in the parking lot. I saw a fading yellow bruise on one side of her face.

I took the change in her mood as a cue to step toward her. "Dawn, if you ever have any health questions come on over to the clinic, okay?" As soon as I heard my words, they sounded lame. Striking up conversations with strangers—especially with homeless teens in a parking lot—did not come easily to me.

Still looking down, Dawn nodded, then turned to the group of men. "See you later, losers!" Hands stuffed into her jacket pockets, she walked off in the direction of The Block. The Block was the name for the perimeter around the main public library downtown, an area known for street prostitution. There were specific sections for white female prostitutes, black female prostitutes, and another section for both black and white male prostitutes, all arranged like items on a convenience store shelf.

The Virginia state laws weren't helping the outreach workers with Dawn. The age of consent for sex was fifteen, and even though prostitution was illegal, the cops looked the other way. Virginia had antiquated but still sporadically-enforced sodomy laws, which defined crimes against nature like oral and anal sex—even between married people—or any sexual intercourse between unmarried persons. The male descendants of the men that had made these laws were now lawyers who staunchly defended the sodomy laws as having "ancestry going back to Judaic and

Christian law." They worked in offices near The Block. Some were Dawn's customers. I was learning these sorts of things by doing outreach with the city's Street Team of savvy social workers and mental health counselors. They were introducing me to a world much different from the one I had known. Through my work I was being exposed to realities of people's lives lived on the margins of society.

In every city, people live on the fringes, stuffed into nooks and crannies, living on the edge of homelessness. Richmond was no exception. There were cheap motels for prostitutes and for homeless people, who occasionally scraped together enough money to buy a room for a few nights and have all-night parties with as many of their friends as they could smuggle in. Most of these motels were sprawling one-story buildings along the older car and trucking routes, like US Route 301, where the Street Center was located. They had beds with Magic Fingers vibrating massage, thin walls, stained carpeting, and leaky plumbing. Then there were the aging hotels, now turned into single-room-occupancy housing units, or SROs. These had once been respectable hotels but were now in decline, their owners renting cheap to anyone willing to pay.

For over a century SROs had filled a need for inner-city low-income housing for transients, students, itinerant workers, artists and musicians, older adults on fixed incomes, and women fleeing abusive home situations. SROs were in aging downtown hotels, which had single bedrooms with shared bathrooms and rudimentary kitchen facilities on each floor. The US Department of Housing and Urban Development policy makers considered SROs to be substandard housing, because most did not meet minimum fire or earthquake safety codes. Most of the SROs were located in downtown areas that were being gentrified, a process that accelerated in the 1970s and '80s.

The summer I met Dawn, there was one main SRO hotel where many of my patients lived. The Capitol Hotel was located downtown near Saint Paul's Episcopal Church and the white dome of the State Capitol Building. City developers were working hard to get the hotel condemned. Many Richmonders considered the six-story Capitol Hotel an eyesore and a magnet for prostitution and drug dealing. A physician owned the hotel. Housing advocates referred to him as Richmond's worst slumlord. He rented rooms for $200 a month and kept a few rooms for nightly use only. He charged twenty dollars per night for these rooms, plus a five-dollar "visitor's fee" in order to get a cut on the prostitution and drug dealing he knew went on in the hotel. Some families with children lived there; a Richmond Public School bus stopped in front of the hotel.

The Capitol Hotel was also a regular stop for the Street Team. One day soon after I had met Dawn, Street Team members asked me to accompany them to check on an elderly man. He was in his seventies and was an alcoholic they had gotten off the streets, through detox, and into the Capitol Hotel. He had hurt his knee and couldn't get out of his room to see a doctor.

It was a bright, hot, humid morning in late August. I followed the two outreach workers up the external stairs, between a series of thick marble columns holding up the portico, and in through the heavy brass front doors. Inside it was dark and I felt blinded, as if a stinking blanket had been thrown over my head. It smelled of rotting garbage, mold, and urine, oddly combined with the sweet smell of hay. As my eyes adjusted to the light, I looked around in search of the source of the hay smell, but couldn't find it. The outreach workers were talking with a muscular, T-shirt-clad black man at the front desk. He was sitting behind protective bars as if he were at an all-night store. A bare lightbulb dangled from a frayed cord behind his head. Old pinball machines were in one corner of the otherwise empty, cavernous front lobby. On the other side of the lobby from the front desk was a caged elevator with a large hand-lettered sign taped to it: "Broke. Use stairs." From the curled and yellowed paper it looked as if the sign had been hanging there for years.

There was a wide central staircase lit by a tall window partially covered by a torn curtain. The wine-colored wall-to-wall carpeting was tattered, stained, and oily-looking. As we climbed the stairs, I noticed thick black mold radiating from the bottom of the window, out over the wall, and onto the damp rug. The smell of mold and urine was overwhelming. We climbed the stairs to the fourth floor, each floor lit by a solitary lightbulb illuminating lines of scarred wooden doors. I didn't see any people. The hotel was eerily silent—no voices, no music, no footfalls except our own.

The outreach workers knocked on and opened a door at the end of a hallway on the fourth floor. Inside the small room, a thin, gray-haired black man lay on a bare ticking striped mattress. He had his right knee propped up on a dingy pillow. He let me examine his knee, which was sprained and probably arthritic. I wrapped it with an elastic bandage and gave him some over-the-counter pain medication I had in my medical bag. I couldn't imagine how he navigated the hotel stairs. He was quiet, polite. His room was littered with fast-food boxes and bags, but no alcohol cans or bottles, so maybe his sobriety was sticking. I wasn't sure I'd be able to stay sober for long if I had to live in a

place like this. I knew that growing old was no fun for anyone, but having to grow old in a building like this seemed
criminal.

After finishing our visit, we walked down to the hotel
lobby. Now that my eyes had adjusted to the dim lighting, I looked around, again searching for the source of the
hay smell. When I asked one of the Street Team members
about it, he laughed and said, "That's marijuana, Jo—
don't you know?"

"Oh yeah," I replied, feeling unsophisticated and naive.

Suddenly a young woman, scantily clad in cutoff jeans
and tank top, ran past us toward the front door. It was Dawn.

"Nurse, I gotta come see ya soon!" she yelled in my
direction as the door slammed behind her.

The next week Dawn showed up at the Street Center
Clinic accompanied by one of the female Street Team counselors. It was a slow morning and no one else was in the
clinic. The waiting room was clean and sparsely furnished,
with a row of orange plastic chairs and a small wooden
bookshelf full of patient education pamphlets alongside
pocket-sized New Testaments. On the wall was a large col-
orful poster of the Twenty-Third Psalm, with a shepherd's
staff silhouetted in the background.

"I hate this place. It creeps me out!" Dawn said loudly
in lieu of a greeting. This didn't surprise me. Maybe she
was referring to our overtly religious decor—what with all
the crosses and Bibles—but I assumed the entire building
disturbed her. The Street Center clients were mostly men,
and the Center had a reputation for being a violent place.
Women and homeless teens might come for a quick meal or
a shower but they rarely lingered.

By then Dawn was living with her twenty-year-old boyfriend Red in a boarded-up building downtown. Red had

been the man I'd seen Dawn pestering on the sidewalk the day I met her.

"Dawn, come on in the room here so we can have some privacy." I tried to sound welcoming but not overly so. She seemed skittish, ready to flee if she sensed fake friendliness.

"Nurse, it hurts to pee!"

I sent her to the bathroom for a urine sample. She had a bladder infection and she was pregnant. Standing in my small lab area, I stared at the blue plus sign on the plastic pregnancy stick, sighed, and walked back into the exam room to tell her.

"No way! NO WAY! I can't be. Red will KILL me when he finds out!" I wondered if the Street Team counselor could hear Dawn yelling and would want to come in the exam room. I wished she would, as I might need help.

At that point I didn't have a lot of experience with either unwanted pregnancies or homeless teenagers. Most of the women I saw in clinic were too old or sick to get pregnant. I didn't particularly like working with teenagers. I lumped them together with mild schizophrenics or drunks: they were unpredictable and made me nervous. Plus, they reminded me of the confusing vortex of my own adolescence, a terrifying time I wanted to leave behind.

Dawn started sobbing, her shoulders heaving. Her crying was surprisingly high-pitched, soft, like a kitten mewing, in contrast to her booming baritone voice. I wanted to touch her shoulder in comfort. Instead, I grabbed a box of tissues on the counter, tore out a few, and handed them to her.

She took them and blew her nose loudly. Staring at the sodden mass of tissues she said, "Red wants a baby, but not yet. We're saving money for a car so we can get away from this damn city. Go to Florida!" Words tumbled out of her.

"OH GOD!" she said, raising her head to look at me. Her eyes widened and her mouth gaped open. "What if it's not even Red's baby! He'll KILL me for sure!" Through louder sobs, she told me she tried to get customers to use condoms but not all of them would. Some paid her extra not to use one.

I sat back on my stool and sighed. I was going to have to test Dawn for sexually transmitted infections, including HIV, and soon—like, *today*. I was mentally making a medical checklist of things to do. This was beyond what I thought I could handle on my own. None of my medical manuals would be of any help, nor would the two male physicians available to me by telephone for consults. This was a complex social, emotional, and health situation all wrapped up together. Plus, I knew that Buddy and most of the other members of the CrossOver board were staunchly against me doing options counseling with pregnant women, of talking with them or referring them for an abortion. I considered pulling in the female Street Team counselor at that point, but decided I should at least finish the visit with Dawn.

"Dawn, it's early. You're probably about six weeks right now, so you have a few weeks to decide what you want to do." I tried to sound as neutral as possible, even though I was really thinking a baby was the last thing Dawn needed right now. As a nurse, I had to give her information on all her legal options: terminating the pregnancy with an abortion, giving the baby up for adoption or to family members, or trying to parent the baby herself—although the latter option wasn't very realistic. As a woman, I had to give her information on all her options and leave the decision to her. But it also brought back painful memories, not only of my own adolescence, but also of my first pregnancy.

I had been a good girl growing up. My parents didn't let me get my long hair cut, my ears pierced, wear makeup, or start dating until I was sixteen, and even then my mother kept repeating to me, "Now remember, your father and I expect you not to have sex until you're married." Within my family I was not so protected, although it took many years for me to recognize—and then effectively deal with—this fact.

I didn't have sex until I was a sophomore in college. My fiancé at the time was in graduate school. I visited him at Thanksgiving, and we had sex for the first time. I discovered I was pregnant at Christmas. I kept thinking of the fact that I had had sex one time and had gotten pregnant. What were the odds of that happening? I took it as divine retribution for having premarital sex and for being in a relationship with an atheist who didn't know how to use a condom correctly. It had to be a punishment from God.

I didn't tell anyone about my pregnancy, except for my fiancé, who said it didn't fit with his plans to establish a career before starting a family. He arranged for me to have an abortion at Planned Parenthood in Boston when I visited him in February. I thought I was in love, so I went along with his plan.

About the abortion: I remember walking toward the front door of the Brookline Clinic in Boston, my fiancé shielding me from the angry taunts of male pro-life protesters lining the sidewalk. I remember the face of the earnest young female intake counselor, especially her long pause and her eyes darting to my boyfriend's when I told her I wasn't 100 percent sure this was the right decision. I remember thinking that it isn't possible to be 100 percent sure of any major life decision. I remember sipping the cool sweet apple juice in a large open recovery room full of women. I remember furtively looking at some of the women who were there alone and wondering if it wasn't somehow easier that way. I remember bleeding profusely while lying in my fiancé's bed in an awful bedroom in a crowded graduate student rooming house near Tufts. Outside, snow lay in black melting drifts. Next to me lay my fiancé, eating a large bowl of ice cream and watching *Hill Street Blues*, a show he knew I hated since it was about urban violence, corruption, and poverty. We broke up soon after. And then I decided to follow my mother's advice and marry a nice Christian young man who wouldn't get me pregnant until after marriage.

I was rattled by Dawn's in-your-face sexuality, coupled with descriptions of her work as a prostitute. When I met Dawn, I was married to Charles. I didn't allow myself to think of sex, except as procreation. It was easier that way. I was glad to now have a healthy, thriving infant son. As far as sex went, Virginia laws made me my husband's property. Secretly, it enraged me to live in such a backward state.

Dawn was too distraught to make a decision about her pregnancy options that day, so I treated her bladder infection and convinced her to let me check her for HIV, gonorrhea, and chlamydia, which all came back a week later as negative. I sent her out the back door of the Street Center accompanied by the outreach counselor, who promised to help Dawn make a decision about her pregnancy.

A few weeks later Dawn had a miscarriage. She came back to clinic for a checkup but refused my offer of birth control.

"Red and me wants a baby real bad. I'll make sure it's Red's this time. Losing this one must a' been God's will. It must a' not been Red's baby, right?" She asked me this as I sat on a stool under the poster of the Twenty-Third Psalm.

At that point I no longer believed in God's will, but I nodded in agreement. Whatever the cause, I was relieved Dawn had lost this pregnancy.

———————

The last time I saw Dawn was two years later, at the end of the summer of 1989. I was out working with the Street Team again. I didn't know it at the time, but I was a month away from being fired from my clinic job for "no longer being a Christian woman with a humble and teachable spirit," for referring women like Dawn for abortions, and for not being willing to call AIDS patients like Lee to account for their sins before they died. I had not known it was possible to be fired for such things. I was six weeks away from becoming homeless myself. I had never thought that was possible either.

Teetering on clear plastic high heels, Dawn was headed to The Block. She had lost a lot of weight; her collarbones jutted out over her pink puckered tube top. Dawn was so thin I wondered if she had AIDS. Lee had died of AIDS just a few months before, so I knew what the disease could do. Dawn refused to be tested again, saying she'd rather not know.

At the beginning of that fall I spiraled down, lost the vestiges of my faith, my marriage, my job, and my home— more or less in that order. My son stayed with his father in the seminary housing where I'd lived as a good Christian wife and mother. So I also lost my son. I spent six months couch surfing, living in my car and abandoned sheds, then in the servants' quarters of the Junior League building, before moving to Baltimore to go to graduate school in public health.

Here's the thing: some geographical cures do work. Sometimes it takes radical change to get your life back. I wanted to move as far away from my birthplace of Rich-mond as I could get. It was a place I found disorienting. Once I graduated, I took a full-time academic nursing job in Seattle and I got my son back full-time. I also met a won-derful man, Peter, and his young daughter, Margaret, who have both become my family, my home. I can now revisit Richmond—for a short time—and not get lost.

In my assembly-line nightmare, my body continues to lie between those of Dazzle and Dawn, but I am no longer mute. I cannot tell their stories, beyond how they affected my life. But I can tell my story.

Epilogue

TWENTY-FIVE YEARS AFTER leaving Richmond, I returned to the corner of Belvidere and Canal Streets where the Street Center had stood. I searched for the remains of my past work with Richmond's outcasts, for my own past as a homeless outcast; I gathered and pieced together shards of our collective histories.

Standing on the street corner in Richmond, I noticed that the empty lot adjacent to the Street Center, the lot that had been a curtain of kudzu vines, trees, and trash, was gone. Traffic whizzed by. Belvidere remains a four-lane street, a major north–south artery through Richmond, with heavy car and truck traffic. As I stood on the corner, staring at the specter of what had been the Street Center, it morphed into an emerald-green mermaid: a large Starbucks now stands there. For all its stamped sameness, Starbucks signals comfort and home to me, since I found refuge in its watery birthplace of Seattle. The Starbucks is on the ground floor of a fancy brick three-story VCU student residence hall on the corner where the Street Center had been.

I became aware of a figure darting between cars, crossing the street toward me. It was Bruce, minus the overalls, garbage bag full of Twinkies, grocery cart, or his little white dog Scruffy. But it was Bruce, still with the same happy demeanor and not looking twenty years older. I had been writing about him that morning, convinced he was dead, hoping he had gotten the trailer he dreamed of living in before he died.

"Nurse Jo!" he yelled as he hopped up on the sidewalk beside me, grinning. Beside us on the street corner was a middle-aged white man holding a cardboard sign, with large handwritten words in black marker: "Homeless Veteran. Anything Helps!" I hadn't noticed him before. He turned toward us. I saw it was James, another former Street Center Clinic patient of mine. He and Bruce were longtime friends, both were Vietnam vets, and both were still River Rats.

I talked with them for a while, imagining this was all part of a Woody Allen movie script. Bruce told me he tried to drink himself to death but it hadn't worked. The VA doctors were good and they were taking better care of him than they used to. He had a room in a house in Oregon Hill and had managed to stay there most of the time over the past ten years. He never got the trailer home he'd wished for. He'd cut back on his drinking and his blood pressure was better. The two men gleefully compared blood pressure readings, trying to impress me. Nurses are supposed to like that sort of thing. James had been living in Florida and had just hitchhiked back to Richmond the day before. He was camping down by the river with buddies, with other River Rats.

"Mad Dog died last month, man. Did you hear Mad Dog died?" Bruce asked James. I didn't know Mad Dog.

While they were discussing Mad Dog and then making plans to hook up later, I looked past them to the south. I could see cars speeding past us on the Downtown Expressway. Under the Belvidere Street Bridge that crosses the Expressway, I saw a group of four white young adults sleeping on old mattresses. At the top of the hillside above them there was a large hole in the fence, and beyond that was a boarded-up house on the edge of Oregon Hill. The Hollywood Cemetery and Confederate shrines remain. Nothing had changed and everything had changed.

The Daily Planet is now the recipient of the Health Care for the Homeless federal grant I helped write in 1987. The Daily Planet Clinic is currently located four blocks north of where the Street Center had been. Next door to the clinic is the same pizza-place parking lot where I first met Dawn while doing outreach with the Richmond Street Team. Several years ago, when I returned to the area to meet with the new director of The Daily Planet, I knew I wouldn't run into Dawn; she had died of AIDS the year I left Richmond.

The Daily Planet Clinic serves over four thousand patients for thirty thousand visits a year. They have an annual budget of $3.5 million, half of which is from the Health Care for the Homeless federal grant. The majority of their patients are homeless. The Planet has primary care providers including doctors and nurse practitioners, dentists, and behavioral health (chemical dependency and mental health) specialists.

CrossOver Clinic (now renamed CrossOver Healthcare Ministry) continues to focus on the 'working poor' with a Christian evangelical mission. The main clinic is located a few miles south of the old Street Center, across the Lee Bridge and the James River. The clinic is in a building that looks like it was a used-car dealership, located on Route 301 in amongst run-down churches, greasy car repair shops, towing companies, and many Confederate flags. In 2013, they opened a second clinic a few miles away, and in 2014, they served around seven thousand patients. Until recently, Dan Jannuzzi remained the medical director of the clinic. He is committed to what he calls poverty medicine: medical practice focused on indigent populations. Myrna, the CrossOver nurse, is running her own Christian missionary clinic in Tanzania.

CrossOver Clinic has an annual budget of $2.5 million, and receives an additional $7 million of in-kind donations: doctors, nurses, dentists, and pharmacists volunteer for Saturday clinics. They call these volunteer Saturday clinics "mission trips that you don't have to leave the country for." A local private hospital donates $800,000 of clinic lab work per year and uses it as a tax write-off. VCU/MCV Medical Center sends student nurses, pharmacists, and medical students to assist in the clinic.

I discovered that Virginia now has the second-highest number of free clinics in the country. North Carolina has the most and Georgia is close to Virginia's number. Most are faith-based. These three Southern states are part of the Black Belt of entrenched poverty and severe health inequities. They remain non–Medicaid expansion states under the rollout of the Affordable Care Act (ACA)—otherwise known as 'Obamacare.' Are free health clinics part of the solution or part of the problem?

Our country's health care safety net is built on the principles of poverty medicine. The deeply entrenched American notion of charity care as the way to provide safety net services engenders stigma, shame, dependency, and resentment among recipients. People do not want to have to depend on handouts, on the kindness of strangers. Charity care further fragments an already-fragmented, disorganized health care system. Clinics like CrossOver and The Daily Planet have to compete for donations, grants, staff, and patients. Charity care further fragments and separates us as members of society—sorts us into haves and have-nots, into worthy and unworthy citizens. Charity care perpetuates poverty. Because of our extreme version of a capitalist economy and the widening disparities between rich and poor, our health care safety nets—whether government supported or faith-based—are struggling to provide basic social and economic support for patients, along with health care. They can't do this well—and they shouldn't have to. Current national health care reform efforts under the ACA don't address these fundamental issues. However, recent (August 2015) federal ACA Medicaid expansion rules allow states to include supportive services, such a housing case management—assuming safe, affordable housing is available. This only benefits people living in Medicaid expansion states, and most Southern states remain non–Medicaid expansion.

I have worked in all parts of the US health care safety net: in federally-funded community health clinics, in faith-based free clinics, in nonsectarian free clinics, in health departments, in the urgent care center of a large urban academic medical center, and even in a private practice whose physicians occasionally provided charity care to long-term patients. Despite compassionate and capable staff and providers, charity care is always leftover care, afterthought care, second-rate care. Charity care gets discouraging, both to give and to receive. As some of my nursing students point out to me, though, right now it's all we have, and for many people it's better than having no health care at all.

In the 1980s, during the time I worked with and became homeless, Mark Holmberg, a *Richmond Times-Dispatch* reporter, wrote articles with provocative titles such as "Homeless by Choice" and "Homelessness as a State of Mind." He spent a night at a Richmond emergency shelter and interviewed homeless people and homeless advocates, who he often characterized as having misdirected passion. In August 2005, when the bulldozers finally razed the Richmond Street Center building at the corner of Canal and Belvidere Streets, Mr. Holmberg, in an article titled "Memory of Building Lingers, and So Does Homelessness," wrote: "It was a sort of one-stop shop—driven largely by love and honest concern—that drew people with tough problems into a concentrated knot of dysfunction."

Mr. Holmberg echoed what many Richmond residents felt toward The Daily Planet, that it was synonymous with softhearted, wrongheaded homeless advocacy. And for the fifteen years of its existence, the Richmond Street Center was synonymous with The Daily Planet. Part of me agrees with this assessment, and I see that I was one of those softhearted, wrongheaded homeless advocates. But I'm glad I was. I still believe it's better than becoming the hardhearted alternative. Even though I didn't rely on homeless advocates or their services when I experienced homelessness myself, the knowledge that they were there helped me survive and move on.

The dark, hulking 1920s-era three-story brick building on Canal Street that housed the Richmond Street Center was owned by the City of Richmond. Beginning in 1985, the City leased the building to the Street Center's lead agency, The Daily Planet, for $10 a year. Sheila negotiated the deal. In 1993 the city agreed to sell the property to the Ethyl Corporation, who offered to pay $300,000 to relocate The Daily Planet. But no suitable site was located in time, mainly because no one in Richmond wanted The Daily Planet's consumers in their neighborhood. Ethyl backed out of the agreement in 1995 and concentrated instead on purchasing the land where the Virginia State Penitentiary had stood for two hundred years. Meanwhile, an anonymous donor offered $2 million for The Daily Planet to move its services away from the downtown business core, preferably into Shockoe Valley, next to the Richmond City Jail. The Daily Planet board of directors declined the offer. In early 2000, The Daily Planet moved four blocks north to its current Grace Street Location. Four years later the City Council sold the now-abandoned and boarded-up Canal Street property to VCU for $250,000 for them to build student housing and the Starbucks store.

Sheila Crowley left The Daily Planet in 1993 to work on her doctorate in social work, focusing on housing policy. As part of her doctorate, she did a yearlong housing policy fellowship on Capitol Hill. Since 1998 she has been president and CEO of the National Low Income Housing Coalition (NLIHC), based in Washington, DC. The NLIHC works on national housing policy issues, public education, and research. They publish the annual *Out of Reach* report, which shows side-by-side comparisons of wages and rents for all US counties, metropolitan areas, and states.

In my conversation with Sheila, she characterized the national policy climate as "a disconnect between the response to homelessness and the response to the housing shortage."

She commented on how homelessness has become institutionalized and taken for granted, with so many more people working within the homelessness industry than when it originated in the 1980s, and with even more displacement of low-income people from housing.

I had been thinking about similar things. After more than a quarter of a century working with homeless people in the United States, it disturbs me that there are more, not fewer people experiencing homelessness, illness, and lack of access to basic health care. As of November 2015, City of Seattle Mayor Ed Murray and King County Executive Dow Constantine jointly declared a state of emergency over homelessness in my new hometown. There are more specialized services for homeless people in our country than there were three decades ago; homelessness as a problem has become institutionalized. Within the federal government, the Interagency Council on Homelessness includes representatives from fifteen different federal agencies related to homelessness. Homelessness has become an industry. There are currently at least one million people working directly with homeless-focused agencies. Homelessness is an assumed aspect of modern American urban life, often portrayed in Hollywood movies as part of a gritty, authentic urban backdrop. I had been asking myself whether by working in the 'homelessness industry' I was doing more harm than good, in that I helped make homelessness more palatable not only to people experiencing homelessness, but also to our housed community members (and yes, even to myself: a literal "I gave at the office" sort of a thing). I haven't found an answer to my question, but I continue to think it's an important question to ask.

Sheila gave me broad-brush characterizations of the Clinton, Bush, and Obama administrations' approaches to housing and homelessness. Under Clinton, emphasis was placed on de-concentration of low-income housing, with the unintended consequence of a net loss of low-income housing units. The Bush administration placed emphasis on increasing home-ownership rates, with some funding going to McKinney Homeless Assistance for housing programs. Obama appointed a great HUD director; Sheila had high hopes, but when I talked with her in early 2013, she felt that not much had been done.

The Homelessness Prevention and Rapid Re-Housing Program, funded through the American Recovery and Reinvestment Act of 2009, appears to have been effective at preventing the worst of a recession-related increase in homelessness, although the numbers of unsheltered and doubled-up homeless increased during the 2009–2013 time period. An increase in federal funding and coordinated services has helped decrease the disproportionately high rates of homelessness among our veterans.

Sheila and I talked about how even the term "homeless" is problematic on many levels. In the United States there have been different official federal definitions for homeless. Until recently the Department of Housing and Urban Development only included the visible or literal homeless—those living on the streets or in emergency shelters. Other federal institutions, such as those responsible for determining health benefits, have used broader definitions of homelessness that included people temporarily doubled up with friends or family, people episodically living in cheap hotels, and people living in cars or other places not intended for human habitation. This more all-encompassing definition includes people who are marginally or precariously housed—as I had been. The HUD classification system was amended in December

2011 to be more in line with this broader understanding of homelessness.

Sheila described being at a Homeless Advocates Group (HAG) national meeting in 2011. HAG is composed of leaders of all the major groups working on homelessness at the national level, including the NLIHC, the National Health Care for the Homeless Coalition, and the National Alliance to End Homelessness. She looked around the meeting room and realized that all of the leaders of the represented agencies and coalitions were now in their fifties and sixties and had gotten their start in homelessness work in the 1980s. She thought to herself, *here we go again,* with the increase in the number of homeless, this time due to the national foreclosure crisis and prolonged recession. We're now past the twenty-fifth anniversary of the Stewart McKinney Homeless Assistance Act, and some things haven't improved.

She was quick to highlight success stories, communities that are pulling together coordinated responses to homelessness with a "Housing First" emphasis (working to maintain people in adequate affordable housing and to quickly rehouse others), as well as a "Housing Plus" approach of providing housing and support services for people whose mental health or substance-abuse issues complicate their homelessness. She mentioned Columbus, Ohio and Worcester, Massachusetts as two examples of successful community responses, and added that Seattle has done pretty well, with a significant decrease in the chronically homeless population (although it increased again between 2013 and 2014). Across the country, there has been resistance from emergency shelter providers and church-sponsored programs, which for the most part have been losing funding for their services. But the Housing First movement has had broad bipartisan support, since it cuts across different political ideologies.

When I mentioned to Sheila what now stands at the corner of Belvidere and Canal Streets, where the Street Center had been, she immediately said, "The only thing I regret about the Street Center building being torn down was the elevator." This surprised me until I remembered what a practical woman Sheila is—a common character trait of many of the social workers I have known. She reminded me that the city inspectors had insisted she fund and install a $30,000 elevator in the building before it could open. She hopes they were at least able to reuse the elevator for another building. She also recounted the construction of the addition on the back of the Street Center for the new clinic space, when a sinkhole opened up in the parking lot. That's when they discovered that the Street Center was built on land that had been the city dump. Sheila said she went back to where the workmen were standing around looking at the hole, rubbing their chins and exclaiming, "It's the darndest thing."

She responded, "Well don't just stand there, do something about it!"

We need more people like Sheila who don't just stand around contemplating problems, but who roll up their sleeves and try to solve them.

I've been a nurse for almost thirty years. I crossed professional lines early in my career. I caught homelessness. I became a broken body on my own nightmare conveyor belt. But they all got me here—to the sublime swampland of living.

Lee, the self-appointed CrossOver Clinic jester, the black man with AIDS for whom I was named next of kin—

Lee got me to where I am today. I visited Lee again in early October 2011 at Oakwood Cemetery, where he'd been buried over two decades earlier. It was a bright fall afternoon, warm and windless, and I needed help to find him. A woman in the cemetery office pulled the crumbling, leather-bound ledgers from a large fireproof safe and looked up the location of his unmarked grave; it was in a section now called Social Services.

"He's in the old section. I'll have to get someone to take you back there or you'll never find it," she said, smiling at me through layers of fake gold jewelry.

The gravedigger was a taciturn, graying black man. He looked quizzically at me when I told him I was looking for my friend. In my Dodge Avenger rental with New Jersey license plates, I followed the gravedigger's battered truck, the bed of which was filled with red clay and shovels. We crossed a ravine, a stream, a marsh. He led me to a wide, flat field without headstones and paced a few steps from a metal grave marker he found covered by grass.

"Here he is. This here's his head."

"How can you tell?"

"They're buried every five feet, heads away from the road. And they sink in. See, like here," he said, pointing to a large depression. "I have to keep fillin' em up with dirt. It's clay here, mostly—not good for burying."

I thanked him and said I wanted to stay and talk with my friend. He nodded and drove away. I was alone. No one was walking or driving in the back section of the cemetery.

Lee's grave was covered with freshly mown weeds— dandelions and crabgrass. Gazing across the expanse of unmarked graves, listening to the sound of crickets, it did not feel like a field of despair. As I walked across the grass, I almost fell into a dark, two-foot-wide hole at one of the graves. I laughed, wondering how I would explain an injury from such an accident. I knew Lee would have found it funny. There was a stone bench to one side of the field, near the road. Dated 1990, it was inscribed: "To our homeless sisters and brothers. Be at peace." I recognized the names of other patients of mine on a few of the scattered flat grave markers. I realized that Lee was surrounded by his friends, his drinking buddies, his homeless family, his next of kin. He was at home. I didn't try to talk to him or make promises this time, but I left some wild asters on his grave.

Sources

THE FOLLOWING BOOKS and articles were ones I referred to the most, or which most influenced my thinking as I wrote *Catching Homelessness*.

- Bauman, Zygmunt. *Wasted Lives: Modernity and Its Outcasts* (Cambridge: Polity Press, 2004).
- Conover, Ted. *Rolling Nowhere: Riding the Rails with America's Hoboes* (New York: Vintage Press, 2001).
- Hopper, Kim. "Homelessness Old and New: The Matter of Definition," in *Understanding Homelessness: New Policy and Research Perspectives*, Dennis P. Culhane and Steven P. Hornburg, eds. (Fannie Mae Foundation, 1997).
- Hopper, Kim. *Reckoning with Homelessness* (Ithaca: Cornell University Press, 2003).

- Ingle, Joseph B. *Last Rights: Thirteen Fatal Encounters with the State's Justice* (Nashville: Abingdon Press, 1990).
- Kozol, Jonathan. *Rachel and Her Children: Homeless Families in America* (New York: Three Rivers Press, 2006).
- Liebow, Elliot. *Tell Them Who I Am: The Lives of Homeless Women* (New York: Free Press, 1993).
- Liebow, Elliot. *Tally's Corner: A Study of Negro Streetcorner Men* (Lanham, MD: Rowman & Littlefield Publishers, 2003).
- Lombardo, Paul A. *Three Generations, No Imbeciles: Eugenics, the Supreme Court, and Buck v. Bell* (Baltimore: Johns Hopkins University Press, 2008).
- Orwell, George. *Down and Out in Paris and London* (New York: Harper & Brothers, 1933).
- Poppendieck, Janet. *Sweet Charity?: Emergency Food and the End of Entitlement* (New York: Viking Penguin, 1988).
- Silver, Christopher. *Twentieth-Century Richmond: Planning, Politics, and Race* (Knoxville: The University of Tennessee Press, 1984).

APPENDIX A

Why We Need the Homeless

AS PHILLIP LOPATE POINTS out, perverse humor and contrariness can help us break through our ingrained ways of thinking, can help us view emotionally charged problems in our world through a more constructive lens. With that in mind, here's why we need homelessness, why we shouldn't be trying to end or reduce homelessness at all, but rather encouraging it. I was influenced by Herbert Gans's article "The Positive Functions of Poverty" in *The American Journal of Sociology* (Vol. 78, No. 2, September 1972) and by Joel John Robert's article "Ten Things We Can Do to Perpetuate Homelessness," published in the *Los Angeles Times* (July 19, 2003).

Homelessness is good for individuals because it provides an education in life not available by other means. If you're young and homeless and have a sense of adventure, you can travel around the country in a Jack Kerouac sort of way, get to see more cities and small towns and different ways of living than you'd ever be able to do if you were not homeless and if you were working full-time to try and stay not homeless. We should encourage homelessness in our young people, as it would increase their civic and geographic literacy and help us avoid the high cost of a college education.

Homelessness is good for our society. First, it is good for the environment because people who are homeless often recycle things. They find discarded aluminum cans and plastic bottles in ditches beside streets and turn them in to recycling places in exchange for money. Homelessness is good for the environment because people who are homeless often leave very small carbon footprints: they usually don't own cars, or if they do, they can't afford the gas to drive them so they rely on public transportation, ride bicycles or skateboards (if they are young), or simply walk to where they need to go. They eat leftover food that would otherwise go to waste and have to be carted off in garbage trucks and take up space in landfills. This especially applies to all of those excess Starbucks pastries that have to be thrown away at the end of each day. Homeless people don't use much electricity, especially if they live outside, and even if they stay in public or church-run shelters, the cost per person of heating or cooling the shelter area is quite cost-effective.

Homelessness is good for the economy because our US market economy is based on winners and losers, the wealthy and the poor: having people who are homeless on our streets—so visibly down and out and poor—reminds us that our economy is working. It reminds us on a personal level that we had better keep working or we will end up like them: homeless. It's a good moral lesson for our children when they are lazy at school. We can point out a homeless person and say: "See—that's what you'll become if you don't study harder!" Homelessness is good for the economy because it keeps coins in circulation—especially pennies. When people give homeless people spare change, it goes to buying coffee or booze. Homelessness is good for the economy because, like migrant farm workers, many homeless people do day labor, such as construction or yard work, for very low wages. This enables businesses to turn a higher profit.

Homelessness creates jobs for people, especially jobs in public health and social work, as well as jobs for journalists and researchers who focus on homelessness. Homelessness and poverty support health care providers, teachers, social workers, and other professionals who are incompetent or impaired, and who wouldn't be tolerated in care settings for affluent persons. People who are homeless—along with other poor people—help support medical innovation, since many of them serve as patients and research subjects in academic medical centers. Of course, these medical innovations mainly benefit affluent people who can afford health insurance to cover the cost of such innovations.

Please support homelessness. Our country needs more of it.

Simple Ways to

Help the Homeless

- Respond with a smile and a kind word—even if it is "No—sorry" when you are asked for a handout for coffee, a meal, or spare change. There's nothing worse than for a person to be ignored.
- Carry fast-food restaurant certificates and flyers with local resources to give to the homeless when they ask for food or money.
- Buy *Real Change* or whatever your local homelessness/poverty issues newspaper is—if there is one in your area.
- Support an agency that provides services to the homeless, especially agencies that also work on

upstream solutions to preventing homelessness, such as low-income housing or job-training programs. An example is Habitat for Humanity, whose vision is of a world where everyone has a decent place to live.

- Be informed and become an advocate for local community solutions to homelessness and poverty, as well as state, national, and international ones.
- Consider joining advocacy organizations, such as the National Low Income Housing Coalition.

Resources to Learn More about Homelessness Issues

National Alliance to End Homelessness:
www.endhomelessness.org

National Center on Family Homelessness:
www.familyhomelessness.org

National Coalition for the Homeless:
www.nationalhomeless.org

National Low Income Housing Coalition:
www.nlihc.org

National Health Care for the Homeless Council:
www.nhchc.org

Homeless Resource Center/US Substance Abuse and Mental Health Services Administration: www.homeless.samhsa.gov

Acknowledgments

WITHOUT THE GENEROUS help of the following people and institutions, this book would never have been written. I am grateful to the organizations that supported my research and writing of this book: 4Culture, Jack Straw Writers Program, the Community of Writers at Squaw Valley, and Hedgebrook. I extend my thanks to the wonderfully supportive librarians in my life, Lisa Oberg and Joanne Rich of the University of Washington Libraries in Seattle. Many thanks to Wendy Call, Waverly Fitzgerald, George Estreich, and Drs. Barbara McGrath, Stephen Bezruchka, Sheila Crowley, and Frederica Overstreet, for reading and providing constructive feedback on earlier drafts of the book. Thanks also to the members of my writing group, The Shipping Group, and to Karen Maeda Allman of the Elliott Bay Book Company in Seattle, for providing writing space and encouragement. A special thanks goes to my partner, Peter Kahn, my son, Jonathan Bowdler, and my stepdaughter, Margaret Kahn, for all their love and support throughout the process of bringing this book to life—and for being an essential part of returning me home.

About the Author

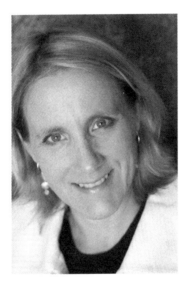

JOSEPHINE ENSIGN is an associate professor at the University of Washington, Seattle, where she teaches community health, health policy, and narrative medicine. A graduate of Oberlin College, the Medical College of Virginia, and Johns Hopkins University, she has been a nurse for over thirty years, providing health care for homeless and marginalized populations. She is an alumna of Hedgebrook and the Community of Writers at Squaw Valley.

Her essays have appeared in *The Sun, The Oberlin Alumni Magazine, Pulse: Voices from the Heart of Medicine, Silk Road, The Intima, The Examined Life Journal, Johns Hopkins Public Health Magazine, Front Porch Journal,* and the nonfiction anthology *I Wasn't Strong Like This When I Started Out: True Stories of Becoming a Nurse,* edited by Lee Gutkind. *Catching Homelessness is her first book.* She lives in Seattle.

Author photo by Peter Kahn

Selected Titles From She Writes Press

She Writes Press is an independent publishing company
founded to serve women writers everywhere.
Visit us at www.shewritespress.com.

Stay, Breathe with Me: The Gift of Compassionate Medicine by Helen Allison, RN, MSW with Irene Allison. $16.95, 978-1-63152-062-4. From the voices of the seriously ill, their families, and a specialist with a lifelong experience in caring for them comes the wisdom of a person-centered approach—one that brings heart and compassion back into health care.

Make a Wish for Me: A Mother's Memoir by LeeAndra Chergey. $16.95, 978-1-63152-828-6. A life-changing diagnosis teaches a family that where's there is love there is hope—and that being "normal" is not nearly as important as providing your child with a life full of joy, love, and acceptance.

Fire Season: A Memoir by Hollye Dexter. $16.95, 978-1-63152-974-0. After she loses everything in a fire, Hollye Dexter's life spirals downward and she begins to unravel—but when she finds herself at the brink of losing her husband, she is forced to dig within herself for the strength to keep her family together.

Uncovered: How I Left Hassidic Life and Finally Came Home by Leah Lax. $16.95, 978-1-63152-995-5. Drawn in their offers of refuge from her troubled family and promises of eternal love, Leah Lax becomes a Hassidic Jew—but ultimately, as a forty-something woman, comes to reject everything she has lived for three decades in order to be who she truly is.

The Butterfly Groove: A Mother's Mystery, A Daughter's Journey by Jessica Barraco. $16.95, 978-1-63152-800-2. In an attempt to solve the mystery of her deceased mother's life, Jessica Barraco retraces the older woman's steps nearly forty years earlier—and finds herself along the way.

From Sun to Sun: A Hospice Nurse's Reflection on the Art of Dying by Nina Angela McKissock. $16.95, 978-1-63152-808-8. Weary from the fear people have of talking about the process of dying and death, a highly experienced registered nurse takes the reader into the world of twenty-one of her beloved patients as they prepare to leave this earth.